Hypertension

For a catalogue of publications available from ACP, contact:

Customer Service Center
American College of Physicians
190 N. Independence Mall West
Philadelphia, PA 19106-1572
215-351-2600
800-523-1546, ext. 2600

Visit our Web site at www.acponline.org

Hypertension

Matthew R. Weir, MD

Professor and Director
Division of Nephrology
University of Maryland School of Medicine

AMERICAN COLLEGE OF PHYSICIANS
PHILADELPHIA

Clinical Consultant: David R. Goldmann, MD, FACP
Manager, Book Publishing: Diane McCabe
Developmental Editor: Victoria Hoenigke
Production Supervisor: Allan S. Kleinberg
Senior Production Editor: Karen C. Nolan
Interior Design: Kate Nichols
Cover Design: Elizabeth Swartz
Index: Nelle Garrecht

Printed in the United States of America
Composition by UB Communications
Printing/binding by Versa Press

Library of Congress Cataloging-in-Publication Data

Hypertension / [edited by] Matthew R. Weir.
   p. ; cm. – (ACP key diseases series)
  Includes bibliographical references and index.
  ISBN 1-930513-58-5
  1. Hypertension. I. Weir, Matthew R., 1952- II. Series.
  [DNLM: 1. Hypertension—therapy. WG 340 H9942591 2005]
  RC685.H8H7662 2005
  616.1'32—dc22

                                                2005043616

05 06 07 08 09 / 10 9 8 7 6 5 4 3 2 1

I dedicate this book to my colleagues, who have educated me on the importance of blood pressure control for preventing cardiovascular events, and, most of all, to my wife, Duffy, and my children, Ryan, Courtney, and Kerry, who have allowed me the professional time to seek answers to the important questions about blood pressure.

Contributors

George L. Bakris, MD
Professor of Medicine
Rush University
Hypertension/Clinical Research
    Center;
Vice Chairman
Department of Preventive Medicine
Rush University Medical Center
Chicago, Illinois

Jan N. Basile, MD
Acting Director
Primary Care Service Line
Ralph H. Johnson VA Medical Center
Professor of Medicine
Medical University of South Carolina
Charleston, South Carolina

Dave C.Y. Chua, MD, MSc
Rush University Hypertension/
    Clinical Research Center
Department of Preventive Medicine
Rush University Medical Center
Chicago, Illinois

William J. Elliott, MD, PhD
Professor of Preventive Medicine,
    Internal Medicine, and
    Pharmacology
Department of Preventive Medicine
Rush Medical College
Rush University Medical Center
Chicago, Illinois

**Stanley S. Franklin, MD, FACP,
    FACC**
Clinical Professor of Medicine
Associate Medical Director
Heart Disease Prevention Program
University of California, Irvine
Irvine, California

Ehud Grossman, MD
Professor of Medicine
Hypertension Unit
Internal Medicine Department
Chain Sheba Medical Center
Sackier Medical School
Tel Aviv University
Tel Hashomer, Israel

Connie Mere, MD
Assistant Professor of Medicine
Howard University
Georgetown University
Department of Veteran Affairs
Washington, D.C.

Franz H. Messerli, MD
Director, Hypertension Program
St Luke's-Roosevelt Hospital Center
New York, New York

Winston Mina, MD
Department of Internal Medicine
University of Missouri-Columbia
Health Services Center
Columbia, Missouri

Ari Mosenkis, MD
Instructor in Medicine
Department of Medicine
Renal, Electrolyte, and Hypertension
    Division
University of Pennsylvania School
    of Medicine
Philadelphia, Pennsylvania

Marvin Moser, MD
President, Hypertension Education
    Foundation
Clinical Professor of Medicine
Yale University School of Medicine
New Haven, Connecticut

Maryann N. Mugo, MD
Resident in Medicine
Department of Medicine
University of Missouri-Columbia
Health Sciences Center
Columbia, Missouri

Joel M. Neutel, MD
Associate Professor of Medicine
University of California, Irvine
Irvine, California

Vasilios Papademetriou, MD
Professor of Medicine
Georgetown University;
Staff Cardiologist and Director
  of Cardiovascular Research
Department of Veteran Affairs
Washington, D.C.

**L. Michael Prisant, MD, FACP,
  FACC**
Professor of Medicine
Director of Hypertension and
  Clinical Pharmacology
Medical College of Georgia
Augusta, Georgia

**C. Venkata S. Ram, MD, MACP,
  FACC**
Dallas Nephrology Associates
University of Texas Southwestern
  Medical Center
Texas Blood Pressure Institute
Dallas, Texas

Domenic A. Sica, MD
Professor of Medicine and
  Pharmacology
Chairman, Section of Clinical
  Pharmacology and Hypertension
Division of Nephrology
Medical College of Virginia
  Commonwealth University
Richmond, Virginia

David H.G. Smith, MD
Associate Professor of Medicine
University of California, Irvine
Irvine, California

**James R. Sowers, MD, FACE,
  FACP, FAHA**
Thomas W. and Joan F. Burns
  Chair in Diabetology
Director, Diabetes and Cardiovascular
  Center
Associate Dean for Clinical Research
Professor of Medicine, Physiology,
  and Pharmacology
Department of Internal Medicine
Health Sciences Center
University of Missouri
Columbia, Missouri

Raymond Townsend, MD
Professor of Medicine
Department of Medicine;
Director of Hypertension Program
Renal, Electrolyte, and Hypertension
  Division
University of Pennsylvania School
  of Medicine
Philadelphia, Pennsylvania

Josh Valtos, MD
Resident, Internal Medicine
University of Missouri-Columbia
Columbia, Missouri

Adam Whaley-Connell, DO
Post-Doctoral Fellow
Division of Nephrology
University of Missouri-Columbia
  Health Sciences Center
Department of Internal Medicine
Columbia, Missouri

Matthew R. Weir, MD
Professor and Director
Division of Nephrology
University of Maryland School of
  Medicine
Baltimore, Maryland

Contents

Preface

High blood pressure, or hypertension, is one of the most ubiquitous yet nettlesome medical problems that physicians and health care providers face in the office. It is an asymptomatic disease, which is frequently rendered symptomatic with lifestyle modifications and medications. However, such modifications can make an individual feel disillusioned and compromised. Simultaneously, health care providers have been presented with new information indicating the importance of controlling systolic blood pressure, particularly after the age of 50 years, and the need for lower systolic and diastolic blood pressure goals primarily in patients with target organ disease or diabetes mellitus than has been the convention. Not surprisingly, this has resulted in frustration, inertia, and disappointment. As a consequence, control rates have not improved substantially. Physicians and health care providers clearly need help.

The purpose of *Hypertension* is to highlight the main issues that we face today: How do we achieve lower blood pressure goals? How low should we go? Are there any downsides to being more ambitious with lower blood pressure goals? What drugs should we use and why? These and many other important questions are dealt with herein by an experienced group of clinicians who have devoted the majority of their medical careers to improving strategies for managing hypertensive patients. The chapters cover the essential problems and questions in a lucid fashion with a nice summary of key take-home points at the end.

The topics and issues are discussed and debated in an open and honest fashion. The authors have been challenged to provide their opinions, not just the "consensus" on their topics. It is to be hoped that this will give the reader better insight and perspective on the various strategies to improve blood pressure control in clinical practice.

Matthew R. Weir, MD

1

■　■　■

Prevention, Detection, and Clinical Presentations of Hypertension

Matthew R. Weir, MD

Hypertension is a level of blood pressure (BP) in a given patient for which the benefits of treatment outweigh the risks. Treatment should be a carefully individualized effort that considers the unique circumstances of each patient. The prevalence of hypertension, along with the complications it poses regarding cardiovascular events, is increasing dramatically, largely because of obesity and the aging population. Approximately 65 million Americans have hypertension, which is more than 50% of the people over age 60. Data from the Framingham Heart Study suggest that the residual lifetime risk for developing hyptertension is approximately 90% and the probability of requiring antihypertensive medication is 60% for middle-aged and older individuals (Figure 1-1) (1).

Prevention

Clinical evidence solidly indicates that hypertension increases the mortality and morbidity associated with coronary heart disease, stroke, congestive heart failure, and end-stage kidney disease (2). Therefore, early identification of patients at risk for hypertension and therapy to prevent hypertension are ever more important. Data from 61 observational studies of more than 1 million patients have shown that death from myocardial infarction and cerebral vascular accident increases progressively with, and linear to, BPs of 115/75 mm Hg and higher (Figure 1-2) (3). Increased risks for cardiovascular events are present in individuals from 40 to 89 years of age. Amazingly, for every 20 mm Hg systolic or 10 mm Hg diastolic increase in BP, there is a doubling of mortality from both myocardial infarction and stroke. Additional data from the Framingham Heart Study demonstrate that BP

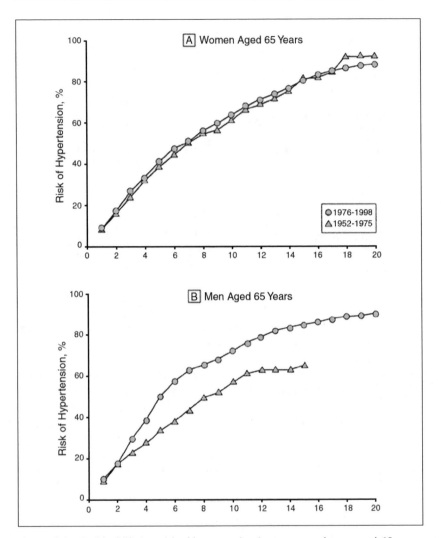

Figure 1-1   Residual lifetime risk of hypertension in women and men aged 65 years. Cumulative incidence of hypertension in 65-year-old men 1952-1975 are truncated at 15 years because there were few participants in this age category who were followed up beyond 1975. (Republished with permission from Vasan RS, Beiser A, Seshadri S, et al. Residual lifetime risk for developing hypertension in middle-aged women and men. JAMA. 2002;287:1003-10.)

values in the 130-139 mm Hg range are associated with a more than 2-fold increased risk for cardiovascular events compared with patients with systolic BPs below 120 mm Hg (1). Thus, a future public health challenge will be prevention of hypertension. If the rise in BP with age and obesity can be prevented or at least diminished, much of the associated cardiovascular sequelae can be effectively prevented.

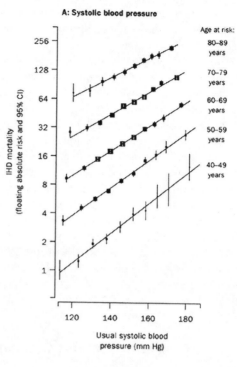

Figure 1-2 Ischemic heart disease mortality rate in each decade of age versus usual blood pressure at the start of that decade. (Republished with permission from Lewington S, Clarke R, Qizilbash N, et al. Age-specific relevance of usual blood pressure to vascular mortality: a meta-analysis of individual data for one million adults in 61 prospective studies. Lancet. 2002;360:1903-13.)

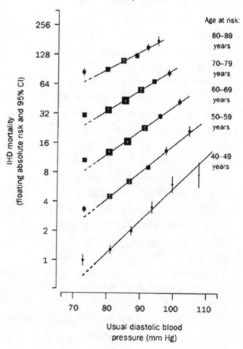

The most important causal factors for development of hypertension include obesity, excessive dietary salt consumption, reduced physical activity, excess alcohol intake, cigarette smoking, and inadequate intake of fruits, vegetables, and potassium (4). Fewer than 20% of Americans engage in regular physical activity, and only 25% consume five or more servings of fruits and vegetables daily. Mean sodium intake is approximately 4100 mg per day for men and 2750 mg per day for women, most of which comes from processed foods (5). A healthier lifestyle could dramatically decrease the risk for developing hypertension.

The major barriers for effective prevention of hypertension include insufficient attention to education by health care providers and, perhaps even more important, lack of reimbursement for health-education services. Many restaurants serve increasingly large helpings and patients often rapidly consume their food, both of which result in a substantial caloric intake. There is lack of availability of healthy food choices in many schools, work sites, and restaurants. Salt is added to food by industry and restaurants to enhance taste and flavor, and foods lower in salt and calories are frequently more expensive. These factors confound public health, clinician, and patient efforts to reduce BP through diet.

Definition and Clinical Presentation

Substantial efforts have been made recently to define hypertension. National guidelines are published every few years and can be adopted on an individualized basis for each patient. Because evidence from epidemiologic studies indicates a linear risk for increased cardiovascular events associated with levels of BP above 115-120 mm Hg systolic, definitions for hypertension have changed accordingly (Figure 1-3) (6). Current JNC-7 definitions describe BPs below 120/80 mm Hg as normal because they are least likely to be associated with cardiovascular events (Table 1-1) (7). On the other hand, hypertension is still defined as BP greater than 140/90 mm Hg. A new category entitled "prehypertension" describes patients who are not normal but not yet hypertensive (120-139/80-89 mm Hg). This emphasis on defining the intermediate range of BPs as prehypertensive is designed to alert both patients and health care providers that prehypertensive levels of BP are associated with more cardiovascular risk and that lifestyle modifications should therefore be encouraged. Depending on physician determination, some prehyptertensive patients may even require pharmacotherapy for BP control.

The evolution of guideline recommendations makes clear that for increasing numbers of patients the treatment goal is to lower BP to below 130/80 mm Hg. This is in large part related to the epidemic of obesity and diabetes and their frequent associated target-organ damage. It is not unusual for patients to require a lower systolic goal of 130 rather than the

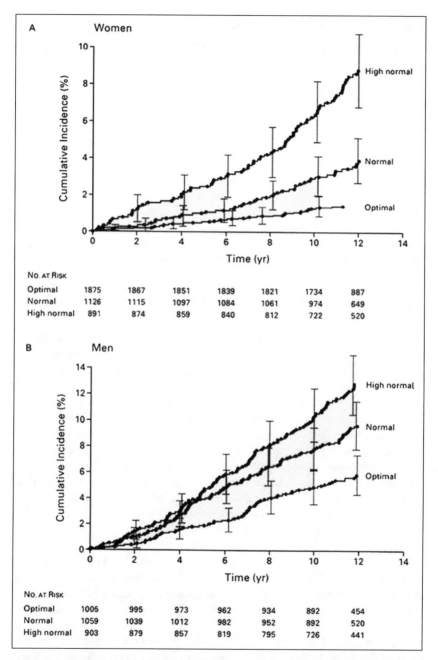

Figure 1-3   Impact of high normal blood pressure on the risk of cardiovascular disease. Cumulative incidence of cardiovascular events in women (**A**) and men (**B**) without hypertension, according to blood-pressure category at the baseline examination. (Republished with permission from Vasan RS, Larson MG, Leip EP, et al. Impact of high-normal blood pressure on the risk of cardiovascular disease. N Engl J Med. 2001;345:1291-7.)

Table 1-1   JNC-7 Classification of Blood Pressure for Adults

BP Classification	SBP mm Hg	DBP mm Hg
Normal	<120	and <80
Prehypertension	120-139	or 80-89
Stage 1 hypertension	140-159	or 90-99
Stage 2 hypertension	≥160	or ≥100

Adapted with permission from JNC-7. JAMA. 2003;239:256-72.

more tradition goal of 140 mm Hg (e.g., patients with diabetes, chronic kidney disease, evidence of target organ damage). There is much more emphasis now on treating systolic rather than diastolic BP in patients over the age of 45 years. However, this is not to say that diastolic BP does not provide important information; rather, with increasing age, systolic BP provides a much more valid measure of hypertensive cardiovascular risk.

Etiology and Diagnosis

Hypertension observed in clinical practice is usually *essential*. That is, the hypertension is probably of genetic origin. Most data indicate that subtle disturbances in sodium handling by the kidney lead to increases in arterial pressure. Approximately 10% of hypertension is *secondary* in nature, which can be attributed to either a kidney or an endocrine cause. The most common secondary causes are renal parenchymal or vascular disease. Subtle degrees of kidney dysfunction are almost always associated with BP elevation. Likewise, renal artery disease can also occur at any age and can be associated with increased BP. Endocrine causes of hypertension are approximately 1% of the total and include diseases of the thyroid, parathyroid, or adrenal glands. Clinical clues suggesting a secondary cause of hypertension include early-onset hypertension (before age 30), sudden development of hypertension, or sudden loss of BP control in patients whose BP was previously well controlled.

Typically, most patients have essential hypertension and commonly have a parent or first-degree relative with history of hypertension. The patient evaluation process helps discriminate between essential hypertension and secondary hypertension. Evaluation should assess lifestyle and identify additional cardiovascular risk factors and concomitant disorders that could affect prognosis and treatment of hypertension. One should also identify possible secondary causes of hypertension such as chronic kidney disease, endocrinopathies, sleep apnea syndrome, or drug-induced or drug-related hypertension and assess for the presence or absence of target organ damage (Table 1-2).

Physical examination and thorough medical history are of the utmost importance. Routine laboratory tests and other diagnostic procedures may

Table 1-2   Secondary Causes of Hypertension

- Chronic kidney disease

- Coarctation of the aorta

- Cushing syndrome and other glucocorticoid excess states including chronic steroid therapy

- Drug-induced or drug-related

- Pheochromocytoma

- Primary aldosteronism and other mineralocorticoid excess states

- Renovascular hypertension

- Sleep apnea

- Thyroid/parathyroid disease

also be indicated. The physical exam should include careful measurement of BP, preferably in both arms and in three positions; examination of optic fundi to assess the health of the vasculature; assessment of body mass index; examination of the carotids and femorals for assessment of bruits; thorough examination of the heart and lungs; and examination of the neck and abdomen for masses or pulsations. In addition, a careful assessment of peripheral pulses and evidence of volume overload is necessary.

Routine laboratory testing, including a comprehensive chemistry panel, complete blood count, and urinalysis, will provide important clues about estimated glomerular filtration rate and the presence or absence of abnormalities in the urinalysis such as red cells, white cells, or proteinuria, which could suggest kidney disease. An ECG could give clues as to left ventricular hypertrophy. A lipoprotein profile can elucidate cardiovascular risks.

It is surprising how much information can be gleaned from the medical history, physical examination, and simple laboratory tests: they can greatly illuminate potential etiologies for hypertension and guide the planning for goal BP and therapy. Chapter 10 provides a detailed discussion on secondary causes of hypertension.

Diagnosing hypertension is not always simple. By definition, BP is labile in all patients: higher by day, lower by night, and it almost always increases substantially during exercise or during circumstances of agitation or upset. Chapter 3 provides additional information on measurement of BP. It is important that we learn more about the validity of brachial artery BP determinations obtained at home, in the office, and with newer technology that provides multiple measurements over a 24-hour period during ambulatory monitoring. There is intriguing new information that ambulatory monitoring, as opposed to traditional office testing, may give better clues about so called "white coat hypertension," labile hypertension, and masked hypertension, which could indicate a different approach to treatment. However, we have used office-based methods of BP measurment for nearly

40 years to determine cardiovascular risk and response to therapy; therefore, before we abandon office-based BP determinations, more information about other methods of BP measurement and assessment of cardiovascular risk are needed.

Patients with secondary causes of hypertension may have abrupt onset, which is quite severe in magnitude, but they may also present insidiously with slow progressive increases in BP. The presentation can depend on the secondary cause. For example, patients with chronic kidney disease will develop BP elevation, which occurs slowly over time or could occur relative to the rapidity of their kidney disease development. On the other hand, patients with endocrinopathies such as hyperthyroidism or pheochromocytoma may develop rapid changes in BP that are noticeable to both the patient and the clinician. Similarly, sudden development of renal artery stenosis can lead to substantial changes in BP. All of these factors are important and should be part of the clinical evaluation of each patient.

Pathogenesis

Changes in BP tend to occur over time. Development of hypertension is a slow, insidious process. We have been taught to wait and to plan for treatment once the BP reaches a level we deem appropriate for treatment. Traditionally, this level has been 140/90 mm Hg. Studies are currently underway to determine whether it makes sense to intervene sooner and thus prevent development of true hypertension with behavioral techniques and pharmacotherapy. For example, it would be helpful to know whether treatment started at 130 mm Hg would prevent progression to systolic levels in the 140s: this information could have an important impact on determining risk of cardiovascular events and on decisions regarding expensive pharmacotherapy.

This intriguing issue delves into the pathogenesis of hypertensive cardiovascular disease. Why is high BP injurious to the circulation? Although not known with certainty, most experts would suggest that rising arterial pressure creates increased mechanical stretch and strain on vascular beds, which results in localized areas of injury. With repetitive injury and subsequent repair over time, remodeling and restructuring occurs, which affects compliance of the elastic vessels and leads to a loss of distensibility. Subsequently calcification ensues. The net result is increasing peripheral vascular resistance and higher levels of arterial pressure. What initiates this process, however, remains unknown (Figure 1-4) (8).

There is also increasing evidence that subtle derangements in sodium and water handling by the kidney may lead to development of higher levels of BP through increasing blood volume. (Alterations in sodium and water handling are likely genetic, and several genetic causes have been linked to specific genes. In the majority of patients, there may be a number of genes

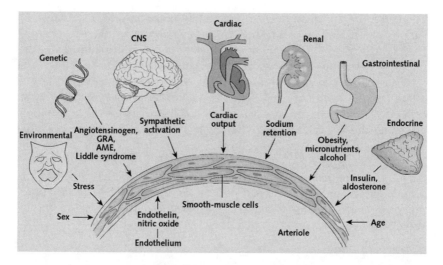

Figure 1-4   Etiologies of hypertension and vascular disease. (Republished with permission from Oparil S, Zaman MA, Calhoun DA. Pathogenesis of hypertension. Ann Intern Med. 2003;139:761-76.)

involved.) It is also theorized that hypertension could injure the kidney and interfere with sodium and water excretion. Thus, it is a combination of factors that result in increasing levels of BP and subsequent vascular and target organ injury. This is also an intriguing issue because it raises questions not only about optimal therapeutic approaches but also about the timing of treatment. As mentioned previously, improved understanding based on new theories of the causes and effects of hyptertension may mandate the need for earlier intervention in order to prevent the consequences of higher levels of BP on the vascular beds and target organs such as the heart, brain, optic fundi, and the kidneys.

Many factors are involved in the injury process. For example, dietary salt is a substantial concern, especially in people who have measurable increases in BP in response to increased ingestion of salt. There are also data suggesting that dietary salt may cause non-hemodynamic injury to the circulation and heart (5). Neurohormones such as angiotensin II and norepinephrine have been implicated in leading to vascular disease. Angiotensin II, in particular, has been identified as a major factor in the injury and repair responses that occur in blood vessels, the heart, and the kidneys. Drugs that block the renin-angiotensin system have a potent capability of attenuating structural changes that occur in vascular beds. The sympathetic nervous system employs catecholamines, such as norepinephrine, to raise BP. Catecholamines have also been linked to the pathogenesis of hypertension. They increase heart rate and cardiac output and raise BP. The impact of stress and hyperexcitability on raising BP is likely mediated through effects of both the renin-angiotensin system and the sympathetic nervous system.

Therefore, there is great interest in targeting neurohormonal systems with various pharmacotherapies to prevent progression of hypertensive cardiovascular disease. Other hormones such as insulin and cytokines may contribute to development of vascular disease, as well.

There is also great interest in the effects of oxidative stress and how it might interfere with normal vascular relaxation responses, resulting in increased BP and localized vascular injury. It is important to realize that there are many theories about the hypertensive vascular disease process that have some evidence supporting them. However, for the clinician, specific targeting of various causes of hyptertension is of questionable importance, with one exception: accruing evidence shows that blocking the renin-angiotensin system, as part of a multidrug regimen to reach appropriate BP goals, appears to make a difference in reducing risk for cardiovascular events.

Treatment

Treatment strategies are often difficult because hypertension is an asymptomatic disease. Patients are not always happy about being told they have a medical problem that could lead to a life-ending event. Many go through a period of denial and are resistant to education and the best efforts of physicians, but it is important for patients to know early on why they need to be treated and what the appropriate treatment goals should be. It is critical that patients understand why certain BP goals are chosen and what is necessary to achieve them.

Lifestyle modification should always be utilized to achieve better BP control even when pharmacotherapy is also required (4,5). Patients should be told that most medications only reduce systolic BP by about 10 mm Hg, which is why they may need more than one medication to control their BP. At the same time, the clinician can also evaluate which pharmacotherapies are appropriate for the individual patient.

BP-lowering medications that are well tolerated and effective make an important difference in risk for cardiovascular events, and frequent use of medicine combinations in single tablets may help facilitate patient compliance. Renin-angiotensin system blocking drugs as part of a multidrug regimen uniformly reduce risk in patients with heart or kidney disease. BP goals must always be met: in preventing or treating cardiovascular events, no drugs are so good that the need for controlled BP is eliminated.

Substantial controversy surrounds pharmacotherapy for BP control. There is even debate about appropriate BP goals in individual patients and how BP should be lowered. From an epidemiologic standpoint, BPs below 120/80 mm Hg are least likely to be associated with cardiovascular events. Yet it is unknown whether it is appropriate to lower everyone's BP to this level. There is also a great deal of controversy about the safety of antihypertensive therapy. Risks and benefits of every therapy must be weighed carefully, especially in patients at higher risk for cardiovascular disease.

Summary

Hypertension is a problem that clinicians face in many of their patients. Its prevalance is increasing because of the obesity epidemic and because of the aging of the population. Hypertension compounds the risk for cardiovascular events and contributes to negative outcomes of cardiovascular disease. Thus, it must be treated. Lifestyle modification and pharmacotherapy can be employed to gain control of blood pressure in hypertensive, and prehypertensive, patients. Research is examining new ways to measure blood pressure, new ways to interpret those measurements, and new approaches to treatment. By incorporating available treatment approaches and the latest guidelines into treatment of these patients, it is possible to lessen, and even prevent, many of the sequelae of uncontrolled BP and cardiovascular disease.

Key Points

- Hypertension occurs more frequently with increasing age and obesity.
- More than 50% of people older than 60 years have hypertension.
- Blood pressure higher than 115/75 mm Hg is associated with increased cardiovascular events.
- Clinicians should distinguish primary from secondary causes of hypertension when determining treatment strategies.
- Lifestyle modifications are critical to primary prevention of hypertension.
- Benefits and risks of pharmacotherapy should be evaluated carefully because therapy is often life-long.
- Primary prevention of hypertension is an important new public health goal.

REFERENCES

1. **Vasan RS, Beiser A, Seshadri S, et al.** Residual lifetime risk for developing hypertension in middle-aged women and men. The Framingham Heart Study. JAMA. 2002;287:1003-10.

2. **Whelton PK, He J, Appel LJ, et al.** Primary prevention of hypertension: clinical and public health advisory from The National High Blood Pressure Education Program. JAMA. 2002;288:1882-8.

3. **Lewington S, Clarke R, Qizilbash N, et al.** Age-specific relevance of usual blood pressure to vascular mortality: a meta-analysis of individual data for one million adults in 61 prospective studies. Lancet. 2002;360:1903-13.

4. **Weir MR, Maibach EW, Bakris GL, et al.** Implications of a healthy lifestyle and medication analysis for improving hypertension control. Arch Intern Med. 2000; 160:481-90.

5. **Sacks FM, Svetkey LP, Vollmer WM, et al.** Effects on blood pressure of reduced dietary sodium and the Dietary Approaches to Stop Hypertension (DASH) diet. DASH-Sodium Collaborative Research Group. N Engl J Med. 2001;344:3-10.

6. **Vasan RS, Larson MG, Leip EP, et al.** Impact of high-normal blood pressure on the risk of cardiovascular disease. N Engl J Med. 2001;345:1291-7.

7. **Chobanian AV, Bakris GL, Black HR, et al.** Seventh report of the Joint National Committee on Prevention, Detection, Evaluation, and Treatment of High Blood Pressure. Hypertension. 2003;42:1206-52.

8. **Oparil S, Zaman MA, Calhoun DA.** Pathogenesis of hypertension. Ann Intern Med. 2003;139:761-76.

2

■ ■ ■

Epidemiology of Hypertensive Cardiovascular Risk

Stanley S. Franklin, MD

The clinical course of hypertension and its complications have changed considerably over the past half century. Before the advent of antihypertensive therapy, young and middle-aged adults presented with severe combined diastolic-systolic hypertension, frequently accelerated or malignant in nature and associated with the rapid onset of cerebral hemorrhage, heart failure, or end-stage renal disease. Although patients do still present with severe hypertension and acute complications to the brain, heart, and kidneys, this occurs much less frequently than in the past. With the introduction of effective antihypertensive therapy and with the aging of the United States population, there has been a shift toward a more slowly progressive form of hypertension that is predominately systolic in nature and affecting middle-aged and older persons. This contemporary form of hypertension is complicated by longstanding comorbid atherosclerotic events, such as coronary heart disease (CHD), sudden death, thrombotic, embolic and less frequently hemorrhagic stroke, and progressive heart and renal failure.

The focus of this chapter will be on the epidemiology and hemodynamic factors that characterize contemporary forms of hypertension and how blood pressure (BP) can be used for cardiovascular risk assessment.

Blood Pressure Classification for Gradation of Cardiovascular Risk

The Sixth report of the Joint National Committee on Prevention, Detection, Evaluation, and Treatment of High Blood Pressure (JNC-VI) and the European Society of Hypertension (ESH) guidelines have formulated a 6-category classification of BP, as shown in Table 2-1 (1,2). This classification is based on the average of two or more correctly measured seated BP readings on each of two or more office visits. Hypertension is arbitrarily defined as a systolic BP (SBP) of 140 mm Hg or higher or a diastolic BP (DBP) of 90 mm Hg or higher. In JNC-7 (Table 2-2) (3), in contrast to JNC-VI and the ESH guidelines, hypertension categories have been simplified with the elimination of stage 3; stage 2 represents SBP of 160 mm Hg or higher or DBP of 100 mm Hg or higher. Prehypertension is a new category (SBP 120-139 mm Hg or DBP 80-89 mm Hg) that replaces the old categories of normal and high-normal BP in the JNC-VI classification.

How Is Hyptertension Best Defined?

Blood pressure is a continuous variable with a skewed normal distribution and without distinct separation between normotensive and hypertensive values. Therefore, an operational definition of hypertension is necessary to identify individuals at risk for cardiovascular disease. It has been suggested that the best operational definition of hypertension is the level of arterial

Table 2-1   JNC-VI Blood Pressure Classification

Category	Blood Pressure (mm Hg)		
	Systolic		*Diastolic*
Optimal	<120	and	<80
Normal	<130	and	<85
High-normal	130-139	or	85-89
Hypertension			
• stage 1	140-169	or	90-99
• stage 2	160-179	or	100-109
• stage 3	≥180	or	≥110

Adapted from JNC-VI. Arch Intern Med. 1997;157:2413-2446; with permission.

Table 2-2   JNC-7 Blood Pressure Classification

BP Classification	Blood Pressure (mm Hg)		
	Systolic		*Diastolic*
Normal	<120	and	<80
Prehypertension	120-139	or	80-89
Stage 1 hypertension	140-159	or	90-99
Stage 2 hypertension	≥160	or	≥100

Adapted from JNC-7. Arch Intern Med. 2003;289:2560-2572; with permission.

BP at which the benefits of intervention exceed the risks of no treatment. More recently, the BP target for treatment has decreased below 140/90 in the presence of other associated cardiovascular risk factors. There is a growing recognition of the importance of "high-normal" BP (SBP 130 to 139 and DBP 85 to 89 mm Hg), "prehypertension" (SBP 120-139 mm Hg or DBP of 85-89 mm Hg), and, especially, isolated systolic hypertension (ISH, SBP ≥ 140 and DBP <90 mm Hg) (1-3).

Prevalence of Systolic Blood Pressure versus Diastolic Blood Pressure

The Third National Health and Nutrition Examination Survey (NHANES III, 1988-1991) showed that there are approximately 50 million individuals with hypertension in the United States (4). The prevalence varies from 4% in those age 18 to 29 years to 65% in those age 80 years and older. Three out of four adults with hypertension are age 50 years or older (5). Using the JNC-VI guidelines to evaluate the distribution of untreated hypertension in the NHANES III population of individuals age 50 years and older, there was a predominance of "up-staging" by SBP (85%) (moving from a lower to higher JNC-VI BP classification on the basis of incongruence between SBP and DBP values) with a 94% accurate classification of BP by assessment of SBP alone (Table 2-3) (6). By way of contrast, in the age group of 18 to 49 years, 64% of individuals with untreated hypertension in the NHANES III

Table 2-3   JNC-VI Staging of SBP and DBP Among NHANES III Participants ≥ Age 50 Years with High-Normal and Hypertension

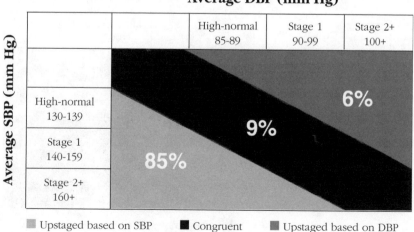

Upstaged based on SBP   ■ Congruent   Upstaged based on DBP

Adapted from Franklin SS, et al. Hypertension 2001;37:869-74; with permission.

population were staged correctly by DBP alone (Table 2-4) (6). It must be emphasized that SBP is by far the most important overall determinant of JNC-VI upstaging of untreated hypertension and, hence, eligibility for therapy, because the great majority of individuals with untreated or inadequately treated hypertension are 50 years of age or older with an 80% prevalence of ISH (6).

Hemodynamic Patterns of Age-Related Changes in Blood Pressure

Both cross-sectional and longitudinal population studies, including those from Framingham, have demonstrated that SBP rises from adolescence through most of adulthood, whereas DBP, although initially increasing with age, levels off at age 50 to 55 and decreases after age 60 to 65 (7). Thus pulse pressure (PP), defined by the difference between peak SBP and end DBP, increases after age 50 to 55, a change that is accelerated from the age of 60 to 65 and beyond. Increased PP may be a surrogate marker for several possible pathologic mechanisms, all originating from the underlying increased central arterial stiffness and contributing to disorders of the myocardium (8).

The rise in both SBP and DBP up to age 50 to 55 can best be explained by the dominance of increased peripheral vascular resistance in individuals with normal cardiac outputs (Table 2-5) (7). Although hypertension in children and adolescents is frequently associated with increased cardiac output,

Table 2-4   JNC-VI Staging of SBP and DBP Among NHANES III Participants < Age 50 Years with High-Normal and Hypertension

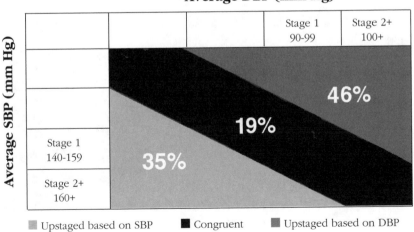

Adapted from Franklin SS, et al. Hypertension 2001;37:869-74; with permission.

Table 2-5   Hemodynamic Patterns of Age-Related Changes in Blood Pressure

Age (Years)	DBP (mm Hg)	SBP (mm Hg)	MAP (mm Hg)	PP (mm Hg)	Hemodynamics
30-49	↑	↑	↑	→ ↑	R > S
50-59	→	↑	→	↑ ↑	R = S
≥60	↓	↑	→ ↓	↑↑↑↑	S > R

R = small-vessel resistance; S = large-vessel stiffness; DBP = diastolic blood pressure; SBP = systolic blood pressure; MAP = mean arterial pressure; PP = pulse pressure; ↑ = increase; ↓ = decrease; → = no change. Adapted from Franklin SS, et al. Circulation 1997;96:308-15; with permission.

the underlying hemodynamic mechanism associated with essential hypertension in young adults is increased peripheral vascular resistance (7). In contrast, after the sixth decade of life, both increasing PP and decreasing DBP are surrogate measurements for central elastic artery stiffness. The fall in DBP with increasing aortic stiffness is explained by a diminished hydraulic buffering system leading to greater peripheral run-off of stroke volume during systole. Thus, with less blood remaining in the aorta at the beginning of diastole, and with diminished elastic recoil, DBP decreases with increased steepness of diastolic decay. In addition, after age 60 years, central arterial stiffness overrides increased systemic vascular resistance and becomes the dominant hemodynamic factor in both normotensive and hypertensive individuals, as manifested by an increase in SBP, a decrease in DBP, and hence a rise in PP (7). Hypertension, left untreated, may accelerate stiffening of elastic arteries, which, in turn, may set up a vicious cycle of worsening hypertension and further increases in elastic artery stiffness.

Characteristics of Hypertension as a Cardiovascular Risk Factor

It has long been recognized that elevated BP is a risk factor for future cardiovascular events and that lowering it may save lives. The relationship is *strong, continuous, and graded* without any distinct threshold level; it is present, in both men and women, in younger and older adults, and in those with and without known CHD; it is present in different countries and in different ethnic and racial groups. The key new message of JNC-7, based on a meta-analysis from the Prospective Studies Collaboration group, is that starting at 115/75 mm Hg, cardiovascular mortality doubles with each increment of 20/10 mm Hg throughout the BP range (9). Furthermore, hypertension is also a risk marker for other cardiovascular risk factors (dyslipidemia, diabetes, obesity, etc.), which generally tend to cluster with hypertension (10). In the presence of these other risk factors, there is a steeper relation between levels of BP elevation and cardiovascular morbidity and mortality (11).

There is evidence of the age-related increase in BP throughout adulthood, so that even persons who are normotensive at age 55 have a 90% lifetime risk for developing hypertension (12). However, the rate of age-related rise in BP varies greatly between individuals. Age-related *tracking of increased BP* refers to the stability of BP over time in an individual in relation to his or her peers. There is evidence of *disparate rather than parallel tracking of BP*, whereby an individual in the upper percentile of BP will have a much steeper age-related increase in BP than one in the lower percentile of BP (7). This is referred to as the "horse-racing effect," there being a close correlation between the speed of the horse and its position in the race. *Lability of BP*, defined as large random variations of BP measurements from one visit to the next, is directly related to aging and to the severity of BP, suggesting that labile BP is associated with increased risk. However, when other risk factors are accounted for by multivariate analysis, risk is largely unaffected by lability of BP. It is the average BP over the day and night cycle, not lability, that determines cardiovascular risk. There are *gender differences*. Although young women have a much lower prevalence of hypertension than men of the same age, women begin to narrow the gap by their fourth decade even before menopause, and surpass men by the sixth decade, especially in the development of ISH. The so-called female protection from hypertension and CHD pertains primarily to young women.

Blood Pressure Predictors of Cardiovascular Risk in the Middle-Aged and the Elderly

Of the four BP indices (SBP, DBP, PP, and mean arterial pressure [MAP]), SBP is usually the single best predictor of risk for middle-aged and older persons with systolic-diastolic hypertension (SBP ≥ 140 and DBP ≥ 90 mm Hg) (5). In middle-aged, healthy populations with systolic-diastolic hypertension, SBP, and MAP may be equal or superior to PP as predictors of cardiovascular risk. In many populations there is such high colinearity between SBP and PP that it may be impossible to show an advantage of one index over another in predicting risk. Only when SBP increases and DBP decreases, as described in most observational studies of older subjects, does the superiority of PP over SBP and MAP as a predictor of cardiovascular risk become apparent (13). The best strategy for assessing risk in this age group is to determine the level of SBP elevation, and then adjust risk upward in the presence of discordantly low DBP and hence high PP.

Evidence for the superiority of PP over other BP indices was shown in the Framingham Heart Disease cohort free of clinical cardiovascular disease (13).

Future CHD risk was inversely correlated with DBP at any level of SBP ≥ 120 mm Hg, suggesting that PP was an important component of risk (Figure 2-1) (13). The Framingham study supports the findings of earlier

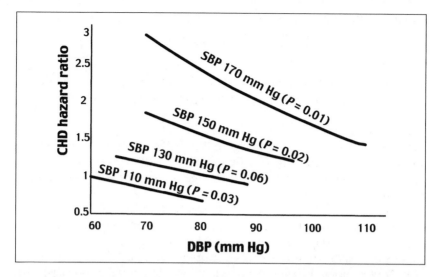

Figure 2-1   Joint influences of systolic blood pressure (SBP) and diastolic blood pressure (DBP) risk. Coronary heart disease (CHD) hazards ratios were determined from the level of DBP within SBP groups. Hazard ratios were set to a reference value of 1.0 for SBP of 130 mm Hg and DBP of 80 mm Hg and plotted for SBP values of 110, 130, 150, 170 mm Hg, respectively. The P values were for the β coefficients for model. All estimates were adjusted for age, sex, body mass index, cigarettes smoked per day, glucose intolerance, and total cholesterol/high-density lipoprotein. (Adapted from Franklin SS, et al. Circulation. 1999; 100:354-60, with permission.)

workers that PP may be useful as an adjunct to SBP in predicting risk and that CHD events are more related to the pulsatile stress of elastic artery stiffness during systole (as reflected in a rise in PP) than the steady-state stress of resistance during diastole (as reflected in a parallel rise in SBP and DBP) (14). At least a dozen additional publications, including more than 15 different databases from around the world, have clearly shown an inverse relation of CHD with DBP so that PP becomes superior to the reference SBP in predicting total and cardiovascular mortality and CHD risk (5). Furthermore, the value of PP in predicting risk in the elderly has been confirmed by 24-hour conventional and intra-arterial ambulatory BP monitoring (15,16).

Secondly, PP may predict cardiovascular risk when SBP is normal or low as a result of ventricular dysfunction. This has been described in post-myocardial infarction, end-stage-renal disease on hemodialysis, and frank heart failure, and is consistent with "reverse causation," expressed as an increased cardiac mortality in association with a falling SBP (17-19). Normally, increased cardiac mortality is associated with increasing BP; in the presence of left ventricular dysfunction, however, there is an inverse relation between BP and cardiac mortality, so-called reverse causation. In the presence of compromised myocardial function, DBP decreases at a more rapid rate than SBP, so that the rise in PP rather than the fall in SBP becomes the stronger predictor of future cardiac events, including cardiac death.

Blood Pressure Predictors of Cardiovascular Risk in the Young versus the Old

The Framingham Heart Study examined the relationship between BP and CHD risk as a function of age (Figure 2-2) (20). From the age of 20 to 79 years there was a continuous, graded shift from DBP to SBP and eventually to PP as predictors of CHD risk. From age 60 onward, when considered with SBP, DBP was negatively related to CHD risk, so that PP emerged as the best predictor (20). All three BP indices in the Framingham study were equally predictive of CHD risk in the transition ages of 50 to 59 years, while in the younger group (<50 years of age) DBP was a more powerful predictor of CHD risk than SBP; PP was not predictive in this young age group (20). Confirmatory evidence favoring DBP over SBP in predicting CHD risk in young adults was noted in a number of earlier large observational investigations and in a study utilizing intra-arterial BP measurements (13,16). These findings are consistent with the NHANES III study, which showed that there were more young persons with hypertension up-staged by DBP as compared to SBP (6). The bias in favoring DBP over SBP as a risk factor by earlier generations of physicians may, in part, be due to the emphasis

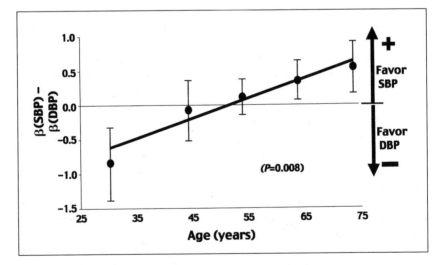

Figure 2-2   Difference in coronary heart disease prediction between systolic blood pressure (SBP) and diastolic blood pressure (DBP) as function of age. Difference in β coefficients (from Cox proportional-hazards regression) between SBP and DBP is plotted as function of age, obtaining this regression line: β(SBP)-β(DBP) = −1.49848 + 0.0290 × age (P = 0.008). (Adapted from Franklin SS, et al. Circulation. 2001;103:1245-9, with permission.)

on hypertension as a young person's condition. However, with the aging of the population over the past half-century, hypertension has become largely a condition affecting older persons with ISH.

Clinical Implications of Pulse Pressure as a Predictor of Cardiovascular Risk

PP is a risk marker of arterial stiffness, which in turn is a hemodynamic risk factor (along with increased vascular resistance) for cardiovascular disease. The totality of evidence supports PP as a surrogate risk marker for arterial stiffness, although at times an imperfect one. Clearly, these findings call into question the prevailing belief that elevation of SBP and DBP contribute equally to cardiovascular risk. Moreover, a high PP could be helpful in identifying high-risk persons who may benefit from more aggressive therapy for control of their BP.

On the other hand, there is no substantial evidence that supports a therapeutic target goal of lowering PP rather than SBP. In addition, we have little information as to the utility of using PP and SBP together, rather than using SBP alone, to classify hypertensive risk. From a practical viewpoint, effective antihypertensive therapy lowers both SBP and PP simultaneously. A public health recommendation that focuses on PP may detract from the importance of SBP in the diagnosis and treatment of hypertension. Therefore, at the present time, it would be premature to modify current treatment guidelines that focus primarily on lowering SBP for the prevention of cardiovascular events.

The Full Spectrum of Cardiovascular Risk Factors

Traditional and new cardiovascular risk factors from JNC-7 are listed in Table 2-6 (1). To the traditional risk factors of age, family history of hypertension, cigarette smoking, diabetes mellitus, and dyslipidemia, have been added 1) obesity (body mass index ≥ 30 kg/m2), 2) physical inactivity, and 3) microalbuminuria (50-300 mg of urinary albumin/ 24 hours). The European Society of Hypertension has added as a risk factor elevated high sensitivity C-reactive protein value of >3 µg/mL (2).

Relative versus Absolute Risk Assessment

The decision to initiate antihypertensive drug therapy for the individual patient remains a daunting task. Over the past four decades, the value of drug treatment has been evaluated in a large number of controlled randomized trials, the outcomes of which have become the basis of establishing treatment benefit. Over this time period, there has been a gradual evolution from

Table 2-6   JNC-7 CVD Risk Factors

• Hypertension	• Diabetes mellitus
• Cigarette smoking	• Microalbuminuria or estimated GFR < 60 mL/min
• Obesity (BMI ≥ 30 kg/m^2)	• Age (older than 55 for men, 65 for women)
• Physical inactivity	• Family history of premature CVD (men under age 66, women under age 65)
• Dyslipidemia	

Adapted from JNC-7. JAMA 2003;289:2560-2572; with permission.

the use of *relative risk* to *absolute risk* as the basis of deciding who and when to treat. Relative risk quantifies the likelihood of future cardiovascular events in a "hypertensive" population in comparison with a "normotensive" reference population. In contrast, absolute risk imparts information as to the expected absolute incidence of cardiovascular deaths or morbid events. In calculating absolute risk, one must include not only hypertension as a risk factor but also age, gender, and all other major cardiovascular risk factors that frequently cluster with hypertension (1,10). Indeed, over the past decade there have been many national and international guidelines for antihypertensive therapy that have used absolute risk in varying degrees to assist physicians in decision making.

Global Risk Stratification

Based on the results of considerable outcome data, there is a consensus that antihypertensive medications should be used as part of therapy in all high-risk patients (1-3). These would include individuals with persistent grade 2 or greater hypertension (≥ 160/100 mm Hg), those with complicated grade 1 hypertension (≥ 140-159/90-99 mm Hg), or those with complicated high-normal BP (≥ 130-139/85-89 mm Hg). The last two BP categories would encompass those individuals with:

- Hypertensive target organ involvement (LVH, microalbuminuria [50 to 300 mg albuminuria/24 hours]);

- Mild increase in serum creatinine (1.3 to 1.5 mg/dL in men and 1.2 to 1.4 mg/dL in women); and

- Grade 3 or 4 retinopathy (retinal hemorrhages/exudates and papilledema, respectively) OR

- Associated clinical conditions (CHD, heart failure, stroke, renal impairment [serum creatinine of >1.5 mg/dL in men and >1.4 mg/dL in women], peripheral vascular disease) OR

- Diabetes with or without vascular complications.

On the other hand, there is considerable disagreement on when to supplement lifestyle treatment measures with antihypertensive therapy in individuals with uncomplicated grade 1 hypertension (140-159/90-99 mm Hg). To date, there have been no definitive trials to define benefit of treatment in this group, which represents the largest single category within the hypertensive population. Ogden et al found that in the NHANES III adult hypertensive population, 20.7% had complicated hypertension, 31.3% had uncomplicated but grade 2 or greater hypertension, 5% had grade 1 hypertension without additional risk factors, and 43% had uncomplicated grade 1 hypertension with at least one or more additional risk factors (21).

Thus, individuals with uncomplicated grade 1 hypertension have a spectrum of one to as many as four or more additional risk factors. Indeed, more than 80% of these individuals tend to have clusters of metabolically related risk factors. As noted in the Framingham Heart Study, clusters of three or more risk factors occurred at four to five times the expected rate in persons with uncomplicated hypertension (10). Furthermore, in this group, it is important not to overlook persons with a cluster of "borderline" risk factors, because they also represent a high-risk group for future cardiovascular events. It is in the uncomplicated grade 1 hypertensive and high-normal BP groups where current guidelines for therapeutic intervention have been deficient. Some of the reasons for therapeutic guideline deficiencies will now be discussed.

Failure to Consider the "Metabolic Syndrome" in Current Cardiovascular Risk Assessment

There is general agreement that people with the metabolic syndrome are at increased risk of developing cardiovascular disease and diabetes (22). Indeed, the cluster of abnormalities associated with the metabolic syndrome are probably more important than hypercholesterolemia alone in predisposing to CHD. According to the Third Report of the National Cholesterol Education Program Expert Panel on Detection, Evaluation, and Treatment of High Blood Cholesterol in Adults (ATP III), the metabolic syndrome is defined as consisting of three or more of the five risk factors that comprise this entity (Table 2-7) (22). Undoubtedly, many patients who sustained cardiovascular events displayed elements of the metabolic syndrome. Confirmation of the frequent occurrence of the metabolic syndrome came from the United States NHANES III adult population survey, which showed an age-adjusted prevalence of 24% (23). Moreover, with obesity at epidemic proportions in both the developed and developing world, the projected incidence of the metabolic syndrome will be increasing and undoubtedly appearing more frequently in younger age groups. Thus, there is a sizable group of individuals with the metabolic syndrome, some of whom may have an estimated 10-year risk of 20% or more, constituting a CHD or

Table 2-7   Criteria for the Metabolic Syndrome (without Diabetes)*

Risk Factor	Defining Level	Risk Factor	Defining Level
Abdominal obesity[†]		HDL-C	
(Waist circumference[‡])		Men	<40 mg/dL
Men	>102 cm (>40 in)	Women	<50 mg/dL
Women	>88 cm (>35 in)	Blood pressure	≥130/≥85 mm Hg
TG	≥150 mg/dL		or treated
		Fasting glucose	110-129 mg/dL

* Diagnosis is established when ≥3 of these risk factors are present..
† Abdominal obesity is more highly correlated with metabolic risk factors than is ↑BMI.
‡ Some men develop metabolic risk factors when circumference is only marginally increased.
Modified from the Executive Summary of the Third Report of the National Cholesterol Education Program
(NCEP) Expert Panel on Detection, Evaluation, and Treatment of High Blood Cholesterol in Adults (Adult
Treatment Panel III). JAMA 2001;285:2486-2497.

cardiovascular disease risk-equivalent by ATP III standards. Lastly, after concluding from risk-evaluation that many individuals with the metabolic syndrome warrant therapy, there is no consensus on treatment. Should therapy consist of statins, insulin sensitizing drugs, antihypertensive medication, or a combination of these agents, depending on the number and severity of specific abnormalities? We must have outcome data before we can answer these questions.

Failure to Appreciate the Total Benefit of Antihypertensive Therapy

The benefit of antihypertensive therapy has largely been based on intervention studies of relatively short duration, which have shown that a reduction in DBP of 5 to 6 mm Hg or a reduction in SBP of 10 to 12 mm Hg results in a decrease of 35% to 40% in stroke incidence and a decrease of 14% to 18% in CHD incidence (1). Trials, in general, tend to underestimate benefit because of: 1) short duration; 2) usual elimination of high-risk patients during recruitment; 3) extensive cross-over from placebo to active therapy during the treatment phase; 4) failure of some randomized patients to comply with active therapy; and 5) failure to correct for regression dilution. Moreover, there are stringent eligibility criteria that result in an enrolled population that may not be representative of the general hypertensive population.

Suggestive but not definitive support for the underestimation of the true value of long-term sustained antihypertensive treatment was noted, not in a clinical trial but in a secular trend study from Framingham (24). Three successive cohorts between the ages of 50 to 59 in the years 1950, 1960, and 1970 were identified and compared for cardiovascular incidence and mortality; after adjusting for risk factors in a Cox regression analysis of the combined cohorts, there was as much as a 60% reduction in cardiovascular mortality in those receiving antihypertensive therapy over a duration of 20 years compared with their untreated counterparts.

Furthermore, there are additional antihypertensive benefits from therapy that escape detection in short-term studies that focus primarily on CHD and stroke events. Effective treatment of even mildly elevated SBP in middle-aged and older individuals, has been shown to prevent progression from grade 1 to more severe grades of hypertension; to retard arterial stiffness and the development of high-risk ISH with wide PP; and to prevent or even regress left ventricular hypertrophy and heart failure. In addition, antihypertensive therapy benefits may be greater in certain ethnic minority groups, such as African Americans or South Asians that have higher absolute cardiovascular risks as compared to white populations (2,3).

Therefore, the higher the absolute cardiovascular risk, the greater will be the cardiovascular protection achieved by effective antihypertensive therapy. With the benefit of antihypertensive therapy being undervalued, the standard risk threshold for starting therapy (10-year risk of 20% or more) may be excessively high. In summary, if the overall benefit of antihypertensive therapy is underrepresented, the absolute risk required for high-risk status will be overrepresented in current treatment algorithms.

Excessive Weighting of Advanced Age in the Assessment of Cardiovascular Risk

Many risk-assessment methods use graded increased risk with aging, which rightly emphasizes the increased absolute risk in elderly subjects with uncomplicated hypertension. However, this emphasis on age may have minimized the risk in young and middle-aged subjects with the same level of hypertension and the same number and severity of associated risk factors that were present in elderly individuals. In this scenario, younger individuals must wait for the development of higher BP, worsening of existing risk factors, the passage of time to reach an older age, or the development of left ventricular hypertrophy to qualify at the threshold level of risk that would justify beginning antihypertensive therapy. This creates a situation in which the therapeutic BP treatment goals are presumably more difficult to achieve and the reduction in cardiovascular risk is compromised by waiting too long before beginning therapy. Many investigators suggest that absolute risk be 'tempered' by the inclusion of relative risk assessment. The Second Joint Task Force of European and other Societies on Coronary Prevention have recommended that the threshold of risk requiring antihypertensive therapy in uncomplicated mild hypertension be equal to a 10-year CHD risk exceeding 20% *or will exceed 20% if projected to age 60* (25). This would appear to be an acceptable compromise for dealing with age-risk weighting.

How Accurate Is Current Risk Assessment for Uncomplicated Hypertension?

JNC-7 guidelines suggest that every individual with uncomplicated stage 1 hypertension who does not respond to lifestyle modification promptly be started on antihypertensive therapy (3). In contrast, the European Society of Hypertension guidelines stress the importance of assessing global risk and then complementing lifestyle modification with drug therapy for individuals with moderate to high-risk (2). This type of assessment requires that the number and severity of risk factors in an individual be used to calculate the likelihood of future cardiovascular events by multivariate assessment, similar to those based on the Framingham risk equations. In the presence of a 10-year ≥ 20% risk, therapeutic intervention would be indicated for SBP of 130-159 and DBP of 80-89 mm Hg. In the presence of an intermediate risk (10-year 10% to 20% risk), consideration can be given for using noninvasive screening tests for the detection of subclinical cardiovascular disease. Noninvasive subclinical disease measures, including carotid artery intima-medial thickness (IMT) measured by ultrasound, echocardiographic left ventricular mass and hypertrophy; and left ventricular global systolic function (ejection fraction), have been shown to have reasonable sensitivity and reproducibility in detecting subclinical atherosclerotic disease. These measures do show predictive value over and above standard assessment of risk factors. Indeed, the Assessment of Prognostic Risk Observational Survey (APROS study) found that 53% of patients previously classified as mild or medium risk by the World Health Organization/International Society of Hypertension were reclassified as high risk (10-year risk ≥ 20%) after finding LVH on echocardiography and/or finding significant increased diffuse or focal carotid IMT by ultrasound examination (26).

However, the utility in using noninvasive screening tests in general on selected population groups has yet to be determined, and no consensus regarding such screening currently exists. Therefore, clinical judgment of the physician and what the informed patient is willing to accept will determine therapeutic decisions in uncomplicated high-normal BP and stage 1 hypertension regarding when antihypertensive therapy should be added to lifestyle measures. In the final analysis, assessment of cardiovascular risk in high-normal BP and stage 1 hypertension is an inexact science.

■   ■   ■

Key Points

- Systolic blood pressure and pulse pressure (surrogate measures of central artery stiffness) are major predictors of cardiovascular risk in people ≥50 years old, whereas diastolic blood pressure and mean arterial pressure (surrogate measures of peripheral vascular resistance) are better predictors in younger adults.

- Three out of four persons with hypertension are age 50 or older, and by the age of 65 more than 60% of the population will have hypertension as currently defined.

- Isolated systolic hypertension is the predominant form of hypertension after the sixth decade of life, occurring about 80% of the time in both untreated and inadequately treated persons.

- Hypertension is seldom a lone cardiovascular risk factor; it tends to cluster with additional risk factors as part of the metabolic syndrome.

- Risk assessment of hypertension alone can be misleading; a multivariate global approach in evaluating risk factors provides the best opportunity to identify individuals at risk for future cardiovascular events.

- It is important not to overlook individuals with a cluster of "borderline" risk factors; these individuals have a high risk for cardiovascular disease.

- For primary prevention, treatment of all significant risk factors, as opposed to treating only hypertension will result in the largest reduction in cardiovascular risk.

REFERENCES

1. **The Sixth Joint National Committee on Prevention, Detection, Evaluation, and Treatment of High Blood Pressure.** Arch Intern Med. 1997;157:2413-46.

2. **Guidelines Committee.** 2003 European Society of Hypertension-European Society of Cardiology guidelines for the management of arterial hypertension. J Hypertens. 2003;21:1011-53.

3. Joint National Committee on Prevention, Detection, Evaluation, and Treatment of High Blood Pressure. The Seventh Report (JNC 7). JAMA. 2003;289:2560-72.

4. **Burt VL, Whelton P, Roccella EJ, et al.** Prevalence of hypertension in the US adult population: results from the Third National Health and Nutrition Examination Survey, 1988-1991. Hypertension. 1995;25:305-13.

5. **Franklin SS.** Ageing and hypertension: the assessment of blood pressure indices in predicting coronary heart disease. J Hypertens. 1999;17(Suppl 5):S29-S36.

6. **Franklin SS, Jacobs MJ, Wong ND, et al.** Predominance of isolated systolic hypertension among middle-aged and elderly US hypertensives. Hypertension. 2001;37:869-74.

7. **Franklin SS, Gustin WG, Wong ND, et al.** Hemodynamic patterns of age-related changes in blood pressure. The Framingham Heart Study. Circulation. 1997;96:308-15.

8. **Nichols WW, O'Rourke MF.** McDonald's Blood Flow in Arteries. 4th ed. London: Arnold, Hodder Headline Group; 1998.

9. **Prospective Studies Collaboration.** Age-specific relevance of usual blood pressure to vascular mortality: a meta-analysis of individual data for one million adults in 61 prospective studies. Lancet. 2002;360:1903-13.

10. **Wilson PWF, Kannel WB, Silbershatz H, D'Agostino RB.** Clustering of metabolic factors and coronary heart disease. Arch Intern Med. 1999;159:1104-9.

11. **Alderman MH.** Blood pressure management: individualized treatment based on absolute risk and the potential for benefit. Ann Intern Med. 1993;119:329-35.

12. **Vasan RS, Beiser A, Seshadri S, et al.** Residual lifetime risk for developing hypertension in middle-aged women and men: The Framingham Heart Study. JAMA. 2002;287:1003-10.

13. **Franklin SS, Khan SA, Wong ND, et al.** Is pulse pressure useful in predicting risk for coronary heart disease? The Framingham Heart Study. Circulation. 1999;100: 354-60.

14. **Darne B, Girerd X, Safar M, et al.** Pulsatile versus steady component of blood pressure: a cross-sectional analysis and a prospective analysis on cardiovascular mortality. Hypertension. 1989;13:392-400.

15. **Verdecchia P, Schillaci G, Borgione C, et al.** Ambulatory pulse pressure: a potent predictor of total cardiovascular risk in hypertension. Hypertension. 1998;32:983-8.

16. **Khattar RS, Swales JD, Dore C, et al.** Effect of aging on the prognostic significance of ambulatory systolic, diastolic, and pulse pressure in essential hypertension. Circulation. 2001;104:783-9.

17. **Mitchell GF, Moye LA, Braunwald E, et al.** Sphygmomanometrically determined pulse pressure is a powerful independent predictor of recurrent events after myocardial infarction in patients with impaired left ventricular function. Circulation. 1997;96:4254-60.

18. **Klassen PS, Lowrie EG, Reddan DN, et al.** Association between pulse pressure and mortality in patients undergoing maintenance hemodialysis. JAMA. 2002;287: 1548-55.

19. **Chae CU, Pfeffer MA, Glynn RJ, et al.** Increased pulse pressure and risk of heart failure in the elderly. JAMA. 1999;281:634-9.

20. **Franklin SS, Larson MG, Khan SA, et al.** Does the relation of blood pressure to coronary heart disease risk change with aging? The Framingham Heart Study. Circulation. 2001;103:1245-9.

21. **Ogden LG, He J, Lydick E, Whelton PK.** Long-term absolute benefit of lowering blood pressure in hypertensive patients according to the JNC VI Risk Stratification. Hypertension. 2000;35:539-43.

22. **Executive Summary of the Third Report of the National Cholesterol Education Program (NCEP) Expert Panel on Detection, Evaluation, and Treatment of High Blood Cholesterol in Adults** (Adult Treatment Panel III). JAMA. 2001;285:2486-97.

23. **Ford ES, Giles WH, Dietz WH.** Prevalence of the metabolic syndrome among US adults: finding from the Third National Health and Nutrition Examination Survey. JAMA. 2002;287:356-9.

24. **Sytkowski PA, D'Agostino RB, Belanger AJ, Kannel WB.** Secular trends in long-term sustained hypertension, long-term treatment, and cardiovascular mortality. Circulation. 1996;93:697-703.

25. **Wood D, Backer GD, Faergeman O, et al.** Prevention of coronary heart disease in clinical practice. Summary of recommendations of the Second Joint Task Force of European and Other Societies on Coronary Prevention. J Hypertens. 1998;16:1407-14.

26. **Cuspidi C, Ambrosioni E, Mancia G, et al.** Role of echocardiography and carotid ultrasonography in stratifying risk in patients with essential hypertension: the assessment of prognostic risk observational survey. J Hypertens. 2002;20:1307-14.

3

■ ■ ■

Evaluation and Measurement
of Blood Pressure

Joel M. Neutel, MD

David H.G. Smith, MD

A detailed historical and clinical evaluation of the hypertensive patient is critical for developing effective treatment. Careful and standardized measurement of blood pressure (BP) is central yet
especially poorly performed in clinical practice.

The evaluation of a new hypertensive patient with high BP embraces
all the principals of good medical practice, such as complete history, physical examination, and routine application of appropriate laboratory tests. A
thorough initial evaluation can eliminate unnecessary drugs from the lifetime treatment regimen that hypertension sometimes requires. Additionally,
it can also identify surgically curable hypertension or other important and
definable medical diseases.

History

It is important to evaluate the severity and pace of the hypertension.
Accordingly, after learning of any current symptoms, the physician should
record the duration of the hypertension, the circumstances of its onset, and
the highest known readings. Was the BP elevation merely on routine examination? Has there been loss of well being, decline in general vigor, or
weight loss? What drugs has the patient tried and with what effect? Has the
patient taken oral contraceptives or other medications known to cause hypertension? Are there drug allergies? Special attention should be paid to potential drug interactions.

A careful review of systems focusing on the primary target organ areas
such as brain, kidneys, and cardiovascular system is critical. Early or

uncomplicated hypertension is usually free of cardiovascular symptoms, but palpitations, increased fatigability, and shortness of breath are early signs. Patients with labile or largely systolic hypertension may show tachycardia and signs of unstable or hyperdynamic circulation.

Headache may be a neurologic symptom of hypertension. Classically, headaches in hypertensive patients are said to be occipital and pulsatile, most prominently on awakening, and to wear off during the day. In other patients, headaches are constricting and non-pulsatile, with either a tight cap or a temporal distribution.

Symptoms of autonomic nervous system instability, such as flushing and the characteristic red face, are common. Some hypertensive patients manifest abnormal sweating, blurring of vision, unsteady gait, depression, insomnia, sluggishness, or depressed libido.

A renal history should be carefully elicited. Evidence of glomerulonephritis, proteinuria, hematuria, nocturia, polyuria, recurrent urinary track infections, renal colic, or renal trauma may suggest a renal basis for the hypertension. An abrupt onset of hypertension at an inappropriately young or old age indicates the possibility of renovascular hypertension.

The possibility of other types of secondary hypertension should be fully explored. The diagnosis of essential hypertension is made only by exclusion, when all other causes have been eliminated. The known forms of hypertension for which causes have been identified are referred to as secondary hypertension. Up to 90% of all hypertensive patients have *primary* or *essential* hypertension: hypertension with no identifiable cause. However, identification of secondary hypertension is important because this group comprises over 1% of the adult population in the United States, many of whom can be cured by specific medical or surgical approaches. The secondary form of hypertension includes a range of kidney and adrenal disease, vascular disease common endocrine and neurogenic disorders, and iatrogenic hypertension.

The most important form of secondary hypertension (important because it is the most common and most curable) is renovascular hypertension, which results from either fibromuscular hyperplasia (usually in young patients) or atherosclerosis (in older patients). In recent years this disorder has become curable with renal artery angioplasty and stenting. It is also important to identify other kidney diseases and the curable adrenocortical (primary aldosteronism) and medullary tissue (phaeochromocytoma) disorders.

Women should be questioned about use of estrogen preparations or oral contraceptives, particularly in conjunction with the onset of hypertension. These are a common cause of hypertension, which at times can be severe, and which is usually reversible on cessation of hormone therapy. The possibility of phaeochromocytoma should be entertained when there is a history of 1) excessive perspiration, 2) palpitations, 3) hypermetabolism and weight loss, 4) tremor, 5) tachycardia, and 6) vasomotor changes in the skin and face.

A detailed family history may suggest a familial basis for a patient's high BP. Also, questions about the patient's lifestyle and environment may uncover hypertensive risk factors susceptible to some control. Obesity is an important factor, and centrally located fat is positively related to BP. Correction of a drinking problem can sometimes reduce high BP. Smoking cessation is important in hypertensive patients, and lack of regular physical exercise may be a contributing factor in sustaining hypertension.

There should also be careful documentation of other medication taken by the patient. This is important when selecting antihypertensive drugs and avoiding potential drug interaction. For example, NSAIDs (including the Cox 1 sparing agents) may blunt the actions of diuretics, beta-blockers, ACE inhibitors, and ARBs. Other interactions may increase the effectiveness of antihypertensive drugs. For example, grapefruit juices and Seville orange juice can inhibit the metabolism of some dihydropyridines, such as Felodipine, by cytochrome P450 enzymes, resulting in significant increases in plasma levels of the drug.

Physical Examination

Measuring Blood Pressure

It is good practice to measure BP in both arms. Normally there should be no difference, but the second reading may reflect a more relaxed adjustment to surroundings. A discrepancy of 10 mm Hg or more should be confirmed by repeated measurements. A consistent difference may signal an occlusive atherosclerotic plaque in the subclavian artery, usually on the left side. If there is a discrepancy between the two arms the higher BP should be used in the management of hypertension.

On the first visit BP should be measured in three positions: 1) seated, 2) after being supine for at least 5 minutes, and 3) after standing for at least 2 minutes. Postural changes in BP are especially common in elderly patients with deficient autonomic function. A longer, wider cuff (19 cm wide) will help minimize falsely high readings in patients with obese arms.

In some instances BP is consistently elevated in the clinical environment, but the patient reports normal BP at home (white coat hypertension [WCH]). In these patients home BP monitoring is very important to management of their hypertension.

Fundoscopic Examination

The fundoscopic examination provides direct assessment of target organ damage, severity and duration of hypertension, and urgency of treatment. The Keith-Wagener-Barker classification system of grading retinal changes is a useful reference standard.

Examination of the Heart

Hypertension in adults is the leading cause of cardiac hypertrophy and dilation and of congestive heart failure. A forceful apical thrust may be found even in early hypertension. A sustained, heaving left ventricular thrust indicates substantial hypertrophy. A fourth heart sound (atrial gallop) may be the earliest sign of hypertension. It is believed to be caused by reduced ventricular compliance, which leads to a more forceful atrial contraction. A third heart sound may be heard in younger patients with rapid ventricular filling. Severe hypertension may be accompanied by aortic insufficiency, suggesting dilation of the aortic ring. A diastolic murmur may be found in older hypertensive patients with calcific aortic disease. A harsh systolic murmur over the precordium or midscapular area of the back in a younger patient may be due to coarctation of the aorta. With this finding, the clinician should compare BP in the arms and legs.

Examination of the Vascular System

Hypertensive patients are prone to occlusive disease, which should be searched for throughout the arterial tree. Auscultation should also cover the carotid arteries, abdominal aorta, renal arteries, and femoral arteries. Generally a diastolic component to a bruit or a palpable thrill suggests a tighter stenoisis.

Examination of the Abdomen

The aorta should be carefully palpated in all patients because aortic aneurysm is a highly treatable condition and often identifiable on physical examination. A bruit in one or both upper quadrants of the abdomen suggests renal artery stenosis. A palpable enlargement of one of the kidneys can suggest polycystic renal disease, hydronephrosis, or renal tremor. Very rarely a phaeochromocytoma may be large enough to palpate.

Neurologic Examination

Gross deficits in sensory or motor function, mentation, or mood are not likely to be missed, but more subtle deficits indicating transient cerebral ischemia or autonomic dysfunction should be sought for clinically, especially if the history is suggestive.

Laboratory Studies

Initial laboratory work-up should include a complete blood count and hemarocrit, a complete urinalysis, BUN, serum creatinine, serum uric acid, fasting blood sugar, lipid profile, and serum electrolytes. If serum potassium is low or borderline, it should be repeated because low serum potassium often provides the first clue of the presence of aldosterone excess. Serum calcium and circulating thyroid hormone levels may point to parathyroid or thyroid disease, which can sometimes exist without clear-cut clinical evidence.

When a pheaochromocytoma is suspected, measurements of plasma and/or urinary catecholamines or their urinary metabolites can be extremely helpful. Also, measurements of urinary free cortisol or urinary 17-hydroxy-corticosteroids can be suggestive, but sometimes the dexamethasone suppression test may be necessary to define the nature of Cushing's syndrome. Determination of urinary aldosterone levels is most valuable for revealing the rate of adrenal aldosterone secretion. This is essential for establishing the diagnosis of primary or pseudoprimary aldosteronism.

A chest x-ray is important in the initial work-up of a hypertensive patient, especially for those over age 40. It can reveal coarctation of the aorta and is useful in assessing cardiac hypertrophy.

A routine electrocardiogram should be part of the evaluation of every new patient. Manifestation of hypertensive heart disease includes T-wave abnormalities, increased R-wave voltage across the precordial leads, which is highly suggestive of left ventricular hypertrophy, and a characteristic strain pattern involving ST segment depression and T-wave inversion, suggestive of more severe hypertrophy.

Echocardiography is more sensitive than an electrocardiogram or a chest x-ray with regard to the presence of left ventricular hypertrophy and enlargement of chamber size.

Renin-sodium profiling and captopril stimulation, renal CT scanning, or renal MR may all be useful in determining secondary causes of hypertension such as renovascular disease or adreno-cortical disease.

Measurement of Blood Pressure

Multiple epidemiologic studies have clearly demonstrated a very strong correlation between increasing hypertension and the development of cardiovascular disease (CVD) (1-3). In a recent meta-analysis including 61 prospective studies and in excess of one million patients, it was shown that for each 20 mm Hg increase in systolic BP there was a doubling of the risk of CVD.

Furthermore, it has been well demonstrated that small reductions in systolic and diastolic BP are associated with highly significant decreases in CVD. There is also a very strong relationship between hypertension and the development of renal disease, particularly in hypertensive patients with type II diabetes mellitus. As a consequence, the measurement of BP has become an integral part of every physical examination in clinical practice as an important marker of pending CVD. Despite its importance in establishing a diagnosis of hypertension, the measurement of BP in clinical practice is neither a reliable nor an efficient process. Measurements are often inaccurate as a result of poor technique and rarely include more than three readings made at any one visit. It is thus critical that clinicians make the effort to obtain the most accurate readings of BP possible in the clinical environment and select the devices that are most able to give us the best assessment of BP in our patients.

BP may be defined as the pressure of blood on the walls of the arteries, resulting from the force created first as blood pumps into the arteries and next from the force created as the arteries resist the blood flow. In one sense, BP may be considered to be simply a marker for CVD. Thus, in our selection of techniques to measure BP we should use the one that is the best marker, or strongest predictor, of CVD. There are three different techniques used to measure BP: clinic/conventional measurement, home measurement, and ambulatory BP measurement.

Clinic Monitoring

In order to achieve accurate measurements of BP, it is important for physicians to standardize the measurement of BP in their offices. The ausculatory method of BP measurement is still considered the gold standard, and the instrument used should be calibrated annually (4). Persons should be seated quietly for at least 5 minutes in a chair (rather than on an exam table), with feet on the floor and arm supported at heart level. An appropriate cuff size (cuff bladder encircling at least 80% of the arm) should be used to ensure accuracy, and at least two measurements should be made. Systolic BP is the point at which the first of two or more sounds is heard (phase 1), and diastolic BP is the point before the disappearance of sounds (phase 5). Measurement of BP in the standing position is indicated periodically, especially in those at risk for postural hypertension. Diagnosis of hypertension usually requires multiple determinations of BP (the average of two or more properly measured BP readings on each of two or more office visits). Based on these readings, patients can be classified as normotensive, prehypertensive, stage I hypertensive, or stage II hypertensive (4).

Patients who are normotensive should be assessed annually at routine physical exams, but those who are classified as prehypertensive and started on lifestyle modifications should have their BP assessed more frequently. Patients started on antihypertensive drug therapy should return for follow-up and adjustment of medications at approximate monthly intervals until the BP goal is reached (4). More frequent visits will be necessary for those with stage II hypertension or with complicating comorbid conditions.

After the BP goal is achieved and BP remains stable, follow-up visits can usually occur at 3 to 6 month intervals, depending on the presence of comorbidities such as heart failure, associated diseases such as diabetes, and the need for laboratory tests.

Home Monitoring

Home BP monitoring, used as an adjunct to measurements taken in the office or clinic, may aid in the diagnosis and management of hypertension. One advantage the home BP monitoring has over office-based monitoring is that it allows for a significantly greater number of BP measurements than is possible in the clinic environment. In addition, because BP levels ordinarily vary over the course of any given day (e.g., levels are higher in the morning than in the afternoon), home BP monitoring, if properly done, provides a much better representation of BP by allowing readings to be taken at different times of the day. Home BP may aid in the diagnosis when there is suspicion that the office reading reflects a white coat affect (BP elevations that occur only in a doctor's office). BP measured at home, in the patient's natural environment, tends to be lower and more representative of the patient's "true" BP.

Home BP monitoring may also enhance the effectiveness of hypertension management. It increases a patient's involvement in the disease process, which in turn improves compliance with treatment. It is also useful in monitoring a patient's response to treatment, frequently enabling physicians to make minor adjustments in treatment without requiring clinic visits. It is possible that the use of home BP monitoring will ultimately reduce the cost of BP management due to reduced office visits, decreased antihypertensive treatment in patients with WCH, and more effective management.

Available Home Monitors

There are three types of home monitors:

- *Mercury sphygmomanometers:* These are not frequently used for home BP monitoring because they are relatively expensive, cumbersome to use, and require some training and experience. Mercury sphygmomanometers remain the gold standard for the measurement of BP and against which all other devices are compared. However, many states in the United States are in the process of having them banned due to concern over mercury spillage.

- *Aneroid devices:* These have been traditionally used as home BP monitors because they are simple to use and relatively inexpensive. However, they are frequently out of calibration.

- *Electronic devices:* These are rapidly becoming the most popular devices for home BP measurement. They typically operate on the oscillometric (perceived arterial fluctuations) method of BP measurement. They can measure BP from the finger (which is not very accurate and should be discouraged), wrist (experience with wrist measurements is limited and not well validated), and arm (measure BP from the brachial artery). The electronic devices that measure brachial BPs are the most accurate of the electronic monitors and have been better validated than the other electronic monitors.

Recommended Home Monitors

The systems that have been most extensively validated are the Omron device, the Suntec device, and the Dynapulse device. The American Association for the Advancement of Medical Instruments (AAMI) and the British Hypertension Society (BHS) (5-7) have developed fairly stringent protocols for the validation of home BP devices. Ideally, only devices that have been tested according to one of the protocols developed by AAMI and BHS should be recommended to patients.

Standardization of Home Measurement

In order for home BP monitoring to be useful in the management of hypertension, it is critical that physicians standardize the measurement.

Five Golden Rules for home BP measurement are

1. Recommend that patients buy a well-validated home BP device (i.e., Omron, Suntec, or Dynamap), which should then be compared with the physician's mercury sphygmomanometer (which should also be calibrated) for accuracy. Machines that are inaccurate should be changed by the patient.

2. Review with patients the correct technique for measuring BP and for cuff placement and ensure that the cuff size is correct.

3. Standardize the measurement of BP at home. Instruct patients to be seated at a table with the arm resting at heart level. The cuff should be correctly placed, and patients should wait 5 minutes before taking a recording. Instruct patients that it is preferable to only take one reading. If multiple readings are taken too close to one another, the second and third readings tend to be inaccurate.

4. Persuade patients not to take multiple readings each day. Frequently they will present with long lists of BP numbers in a single 24-hour period. This results in anxiety over BP and may result in WCH in the home environment. Instruct patients to take only 1-2 readings per day and on 3-4 days per week. BP should be carefully recorded in a log.

5. Strongly persuade patients not to leave out the 'bad readings.' Sometimes they will measure 10-12 readings per day and only record the better readings to avoid changes in medication.

Ambulatory Monitoring

Ambulatory BP monitoring (ABPM) permits multiple readings to be taken during the course of 24-hour periods, with measurements made during the patient's normal activities. Since the development of ABPM, its use has been almost entirely confined to clinical research studies. However, over the past few years, there has been increasing interest in ABPM in clinical practice. Several studies show that it better predicts pending CVD than home or office BP measurement, and that it represents the most reliable method for hypertension diagnosis.

Interest is likely to increase even more dramatically over the next few years as a result of increased understanding of ABPM's diagnostic value and because several insurance companies now provide some reimbursement for ABPM in patients suspected to have WCH.

Devices

Ambulatory BP monitors are automated and programmable devices that detect BP by ausculatory method or oscillometric route, and some devices use both techniques. The ausculatory devices employ the use of a microphone to detect Korotkoff sounds, but unfortunately ausculatory devices are sensitive to external artifact noise so may be less precise in obese individuals. In some devices this can be overcome by synchronizing the Korotkoff sound with the R-wave of the electrocardiogram (ECG gating). The oscillometric technique is less affected by external artifact because it detects initial and maximal brachial arterial vibrations or the mean arterial BP. The systolic and diastolic BP values are actually computed via set algorithm. Hence, the more sensitive the algorithm, the more accurate the device.

The modern ABPM machines are compact, lightweight monitors that are easily worn by patients. They can be programmed to take BP readings at various intervals, e.g., every 20 minutes during the day and every 30 minutes at night. Some devices have the ability to learn the patient's systolic BP and will inflate to 20 mm Hg above systolic BP, which is useful because it decreases discomfort. In most devices the bleed rates of deflation of the cuff and maximal inflation pressures can be programmed. Some of the devices have a patient-initiated event button, which is useful because it can be used to assess whether symptoms can be correlated to changes in BP (either hypertension or hypotension).

ABPM should be performed during a patient's typical working day, and the patient should be encouraged to have as normal of a day as possible. The patient should be told to hold the arm motionless during the actual inflation of the cuff. This increases the speed of the reading and decreases artifactual readings. Patients should also be informed to avoid excessive physical activity.

Uses

ABPM is used to diagnose white coat hypertension (WCH), orthostatic hypertension, and autonomic dysfunction, and to detect BP variability associated with target organ damage. ABPM is also helpful in guiding treatment decisions by providing evidence of patient response to treatment.

DIAGNOSIS OF WHITE COAT HYPERTENSION

ABPM is extremely useful in patients with suspected WCH to determine whether BP in the clinic environment is truly normal. WCH may be suspected when at least two home measurements of BP are lower than readings done in the clinic setting. There is still much debate on the prognostic importance of identifying WCH and whether patients with this condition are at an increased risk of developing CVD. Data from several studies would suggest that WCH may be considered prehypertensive and at some point may require therapy (8-10). It must be emphasized that repeat monitoring is important in patients with WCH at 1-2 year intervals to ensure that these patients do not become overt hypertensives. Frequently, patients are labeled as WCH and it is believed that they can never develop true hypertension. This is incorrect: patients with WCH develop true hypertension at least as frequently as normotensives and may go on to develop true hypertension as they age.

It is also important to assess the 'length of time' spent hypertensive by WCH patients. This is calculated by determining the percentage of readings above 140/90 mm Hg during the day and readings above 120/80 mm Hg during sleep. This measurement is called BP load. BP load is correlated closely with target organ damage. Studies have shown that when patients have a BP load of more than 30% they are at increased risk for CVD and should probably receive antihypertensive treatment.

ASSESSMENT OF CIRCADIAN RHYTHM

The use of ABPM has shown that BP has a very definite and reproducible circadian pattern over 24 hours (11-13). This circadian rhythm occurs in both normotensive and hypertensive patients; in hypertension patients, this pattern is the same as that for persons with normal BP but is shifted upward in a parallel manner. BP is at it highest level during the day. It starts to decrease in the early evening, usually coinciding with the end of the working day. It reaches its nadir between midnight and 2 a.m. BP then starts to increase during arousal from sleep at approximately 4 a.m. and then ascends rapidly from the low nighttime values to the higher daytime values between 4 a.m. and 12 noon (13). There has been significant interest in this rapid early morning BP surge because it coincides with the peak incidence of strokes and myocardial infarctions (14-18).

Patients that have the typical circadian pattern in which BP 'drops' at night are referred to as 'dippers.' The nighttime BP in dippers typically decreases 10%-20% compared with their awake BP, and such decreases are considered normal. Some patients have an exaggerated drop in nocturnal BPs of more than 20%; these patients have been referred to as extreme dippers and tend to have more ischemic lesions on magnetic resonance imaging of the brain compared with dippers (19). Approximately 10%-30% of patients do not 'dip' their BP during sleep, and these patients are referred to as 'non-dippers.' The non-dipping pattern is often associated with secondary hypertension and also occurs in patients with autonomic dysfunction. Studies have shown a much greater incidence of CVD in patients who are non-dippers compared to dippers with similar BPs (19,20). Reverse dipping, in which BPs are slightly higher at night then during the day, are seen in a small percentage of patients (21).

MANAGEMENT OF HYPERTENSION

ABPM is the most accurate method of diagnosing hypertension, but it also provides the most efficient way of achieving treatment success in hypertensive patients. Because it provides more thorough information than clinic monitoring, it is better at assessing patient response to therapy, and may therefore be instrumental in guiding and modifying treatment. For example, ABPM is useful in patients who are receiving what the physician believes is effective treatment but not achieving the expected response. A large percentage of patients develop WCH even while receiving antihypertensive therapy. Physicians may unnecessarily increase the dosage of antihypertensive medication in these patients if the WCH remains undetected. As we have discussed, ABPM is an excellent means of identifying WCH, and therefore may aid in determining appropriate treatment, which in some case may even be to decrease medication dosage.

Monitoring the circadian pattern may also help clinicians make treatment adjustments. It should be remembered that the circadian pattern for BP seen in normotensive subjects also occurs in hypertensive patients but is shifted upwards in a parallel fashion. When treating hypertensive patients, the best result in BP reduction would be a parallel shift downward of the curve throughout the 24-hour interval into the normotensive range. It is important that the reduction of BP is smooth and persists throughout the dosing interval, including the last 4 hours of the dosing interval. Because recent studies have shown an increased risk of CVD associated with a steeper rise of BP in the morning period, attempts have been made to decrease the rise rate of BP (to flatten) in the early morning (22). However, this has proven difficult to achieve in the clinical setting.

Duration of action of antihypertensive medications may be assessed through the use of ABPM. It is clear that once-a-day medication in the management of hypertension enhances patient compliance. As a result, pharmaceutical companies have tried to assist physicians by developing antihypertensive agents that can be dosed once daily. However, this has created a new problem for physicians because several of the antihypertensive agents marketed as once-a-day drugs do not provide true 24-hour BP control (26). Thus, in some cases, drugs dosed in the morning will lose efficacy in the final 4-6 hours of the dosing interval. This coincides with the early morning surge in BP and the time of peak cardiovascular events. It is believed, although not proven, that this is the time of the day that effective BP control is highly desirable. Thus, it is important in the selection of agents to use those which provide a consistent reduction in BP throughout the dosing interval. ABPM is extremely useful in ensuring that selected antihypertensive agents provide smooth and consistent BP reduction throughout the day.

Loss of early morning BP control is frequently missed by physicians because BP is normally assessed at the peak of dose in the office environment, and in this setting even shorter-acting drugs will appear effective. Patients often have the habit of measuring their own BPs at home before dosing. They will frequently claim that their BP is highest in the morning. This is also a good indicator to physicians that the agent they are using is not providing 24-hour BP control. In the absence of ABPM or home monitoring, physicians should measure trough BP to ensure 24-hour BP control. This can be achieved by simply directing patients to omit their dose on the morning of a clinic visit, which should occur 24-25 hours after their previous day's dose. If BP is controlled at this time, the drug is probably providing 24-hour control. If BP is not controlled, the drug should be substituted for a true 24-hour agent or should be dosed twice daily.

DIAGNOSIS OF ORTHOSTATIC HYPERTENSION

ABPM machines, particularly those with manual initiate buttons, are useful in assessing patients with dizziness who are suspected of having orthostatic hypertension. Patients can be instructed to press the self-inflate button during periods of dizziness to assess if dizziness coincides with hypotension. Also, ABPM can be used to isolate hypertension as a result of over-treatment.

DIAGNOSIS OF AUTONOMIC DYSFUNCTION

Patients with autonomic dysfunction, which is not uncommon in diabetics, may have periods of significantly increased BP, which frequently occur at similar times of the day and can be documented with ABPM. This data frequently assists physicians in selecting appropriate treatment for these patients. Episodes of hypotension can also occur in these patients and can be isolated on ABPM. Episodic hypertension, such as that which may occur in patients with phaeochromocytoma, can also be isolated on ABPM.

DETECTION OF BLOOD PRESSURE VARIABILITY

ABPM is useful to determine BP variability over the 24-hour period. This may have some clinical relevance in that it has been shown that BP variability correlates closely with target organ damage (24). Attempts can be made to smooth BP during antihypertensive treatment. It should be remembered that it is a normal physiologic reaction to increase BP in response to appropriate stressful circumstances. This is not abnormal and should be differentiated from BP variability or lability, which occurs frequently throughout a 24-hour period often without reason and is associated with target organ damage.

Reproducibility

The majority of clinical trials conducted to evaluate ambulatory BP reproducibility confirm both superior short-term (less than 1 year) and long-term (longer than 1 year) reproducibility of ABPM compared with clinical BP measurement (25-27). In the HARVEST study, 508 subjects were evaluated; ABPM was conducted at baseline and 3 months later in the untreated state. A very modest difference (-0.4/-0.7 mm Hg) in the two sequential ABPMs for the group was observed, which was less than that seen for the variation in office-measured BP. A sub-study from the SYST-EUR trial evaluated 112 patients who were randomized to receive placebo (25). Clinic and ABPM readings were done at baseline and were repeated after 1 month in 51 subjects and at 1 year in 112 patients. The results indicated that differences in 24-hour ambulatory systolic BP (2.4 + 10.7 mm Hg) were far less than for clinical systolic BP (6.6 + 15.9 mm Hg) taken at 1 year.

Normal Values

Because ABPM is still a relatively new technique there is still some disagreement regarding the true normal values for various monitoring periods. It is also likely, as is the case with office values, that these normal values will change as we accumulate more epidemiologic data. Table 3-1 demonstrates the current suggested normal values for ABPM and for BP load compiled from the currently available data.

Coverage and Billing

Section 50-42 of the Medicare Coverage Issues Manual has been revised to change the coverage status of ABPM from non-covered to covered and to clarify the conditions under which ABPM is covered.

Table 3-1   Average Ambulatory Blood Pressure and Load: Suggested Upper Limits of Normal

BP Measurement	Probably Normal	Borderline	Probably Abnormal
Systolic Average			
Awake	<135	135-140	>140
Asleep	<120	120-125	>125
24-Hour	<130	130-135	>135
Diastolic Average			
Awake	<85	85-90	>90
Asleep	<75	75-80	>80
24-Hour	<80	80-85	>85
Systolic Load (%)			
Awake	<15	15-30	>30
Asleep	<15	15-30	>30
Diastolic Load (%)			
Awake	<15	15-30	>30
Asleep	<15	15-30	>30

COVERAGE

ABPM involves use of a noninvasive device to measure BP in 24-hour cycles. These 24-hour measurements are stored in the device and are later interpreted at the physician's office. ABPM must be performed for at least 24 hours to meet coverage criteria. Payment is not allowed for institutionalized beneficiaries. Effective April 1, 2002, ABPM is covered for those beneficiaries with suspected WCH. Suspected WCH is defined as:

- Office BP less than 140/90 mm Hg on at least three separate clinic/office visits with two separate measurements made at each visit;
- At least two documented separate BP measurements taken outside the office that are less than 140/90 mm Hg; and
- No evidence of end-organ damage.

ABPM is not covered for any other uses. In the rare circumstance that ABPM needs to be performed more than once in a beneficiary, the qualifying criteria described above must be met for each subsequent ABPM test.

CARRIER BILLING INSTRUCTIONS

Applicable HCPCS Codes:

- 93784: ABPM, utilizing a system such as magnetic tape and/or computer disk, for 24 hours or longer, including recording, scanning analysis, interpretation and report.
- 93786: ABPM, utilizing a system such as magnetic tape and/or computer disk, for 24 hours or longer; recording only.
- 93790: ABPM, utilizing a system such as magnetic tape and/or computer disk, for 24 hours or longer; physician review with interpretation and report.
- 93788: ABPM, utilizing a system such as magnetic tape and/or computer disk, for 24 hours or longer; scanning analysis with report; **not** approved for Medicare payment.

Payment Requirements

Payment and pricing information will be on the April update of the Medicare Physician Fee Schedule Database (MPFSDB). Payment for ABPM is based on the Medicare Physician Fee Schedule. Deductible and coinsurance apply. Claims from physicians or other practitioners where assignment was not taken are subject to the Medicare limiting charge.

Costs

Although using ABPM may initially increase the cost of treating hypertension, it has been estimated that over a period of 3-5 years the money saved by excluding WHC from treatment and thus decreasing medication cost as well as a likely reduction in office visits would offset the cost of the ABPMs.

Within 5 years the cost of treating hypertension using ABPM would be cheaper than using only office BPs.

Comparison of Blood Pressure Measurement Techniques

Several studies have attempted to assess which BP measuring techniques are the best predictors of target organ damage in hypertensive patients. The results will help determine the best technique for BP measurement in the clinical and research settings. Home BP monitoring, if properly performed, is a better predictor of pending CVD than conventionally measured BP. There are two studies that have shown that the correlation between echocardiographically determined left ventricular hypertrophy (LVH) and BP is better for home than for clinic readings (28,29). A third study found that target organ damage was less pronounced in patients whose home pressure was low in relation to the clinic pressure than in those whom it was high. In another study assessing the effects of antihypertensive treatment on the regression of LVH in hypertensive subjects, it was shown that the changes in home BP correlated more closely with regression in LVH than with changes in clinic BP (30). Only one, a prospective study of 1789 patients, has published data on the prognostic value of home BP monitoring. All patients were evaluated with clinic, home, and ambulatory readings. The survival rate was significantly lower for people whose initial home BP was above 138/83 mm Hg; however, the consequences of high clinic pressure were far less clear (see Table 3-2 and Figure 3-1) (31-33).

Ambulatory versus Clinic Monitoring

There have been more than 6000 patients in outcomes studies that included ABPM. These studies clearly show that ABPM is a strong predictor of pending CVD, and a better predictor of pending CVD than the average of two or more office readings measured on at least two occasions. A recent outcomes study

Table 3-2   Correlation Between Measures of Target Organ Damage and Blood Pressure Measured at Home or in Clinic

Reference No.	Measure of TOD	Clinic		Home	
		SBP	DBP	SBP	SBP
28	LV mass	0.22	0.07	0.45	0.40
29	LV mass	0.30	—	0.41	—
30	Combined	0.42	0.34	0.42	0.33

TOD = target organ damage; LV = left ventricular; SBP = systolic blood pressure; DBP = diastolic blood pressure.

using a Cox proportional hazards model showed that higher mean values for 24-hour ambulatory systolic and diastolic BP were independent risk factors for new cardiovascular events. The model was adjusted for age, sex, smoking status, presence or absence of diabetes, serum cholesterol concentrations, body mass index, use or non-use of lipid-lowering drugs, the presence or absence of a history of CV events, and BP measured at the physician's office (Table 3-3) (34). It also demonstrated that ABPM was a stronger predictor of pending CVD than office BP (mean of three sphygmomanometric readings in the seated position after a 5-minute rest period) after having corrected for the classic cardiovascular risk factors (Tables 3-3 and 3-4).

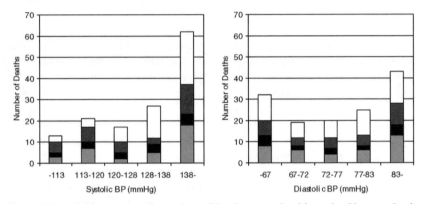

Figure 3-1   Death rate according to home blood pressure level from the Ohasama Study. Shaded bars = cerebrovascular disease; striped bars = heart disease; solid bars = cancer; open bars = other causes.

Table 3-3   Relative Risks Associated with Ambulatory BP Measurements after Additional Adjustment for Office BP at Entry

Blood Pressure Measurement	*Fatal or Non-Fatal Myocardial Infarction or Stroke (N=77)* *Relative Risk (95% Confidence Interval)*
Systolic	
24-Hour	1.52 (1.16-2.00)
Daytime	1.56 (1.19-2.05)
Nighttime	1.25 (0.97-1.67)
Diastolic	
24-Hour	1.41 (1.08-1.85)
Daytime	1.41 (1.11-1.92)
Nighttime	1.25 (0.96-1.64)

Relative risks are for each I-SD increment in BP and were adjusted for age, BMI, smoking status, diabetes, cholesterol, lipid-lowering drugs, CV complications at entry, and office BP.

Adapted from Clement DL, De Buyzere ML, De Bacquer DA, de Leeuw PW, Duprez DA, Fagard RH, Gheeraert PJ, Missault LH, Braun JJ, Six RO, Van Der Niepen P, O'Brien E; Office versus Ambulatory Pressure Study Investigators. Prognostic value of ambulatory blood-pressure recordings in patients with treated hypertension. N Engl J Med. 2003 Jun 12;348(24):2407-2415.

Table 3-4   Relative Risks Associated with Office and Ambulatory Measurements of Systolic and Diastolic Blood Pressure at Entry*

Blood Pressure Measurement	Fatal or Non-Fatal Myocardial Infarction or Stroke (N = 77) Relative Risk (95% Confidence Interval)
Systolic	
Office	1.22 (0.95-1.59)
24-Hour	1.51 (1.19-1.92)
Daytime	1.54 (1.21-1.96)
Nighttime	1.30 (1.03-1.65)
Diastolic	
Office	1.14 (0.86-1.52)
24-Hour	1.41 (1.10-1.80)
Daytime	1.45 (1.13-1.86
Nighttime	1.28 (0.99-1.65)

* Relative risks are for each 1-SD increment in BP and are adjusted for age, sex, BMI, smoking status, diabetes, cholesterol, lipid lowering agents, and CV complications at entry.
Adapted from Clement DL, De Buyzere ML, De Bacquer DA, et al. Prognostic value of ambulatory blood-pressure recordings in patients with treated hypertension. N Engl J Med. 2003;348:2407-15; with permission.

In a sub-study of the Systolic Hypertension in Europe (Syst-Eur) Trial, 808 patients (age older than 60 years) whose untreated systolic BP level on conventional measurements at baseline was 160-219 mm Hg and whose baseline diastolic BP was under 95 mm Hg were subjected to ABPM (35). A mean of six conventional sphygmomanometer readings (two measurements in the sitting position at three visits 1 month apart) constitutes the value for the office reading. The study was started in October 1985 with follow-up until February 1999. Study end-points were total CV mortality, all CV end-points, fatal and non-fatal stroke, and fatal and non-fatal cardiac end-points. The study clearly demonstrated that ambulatory systolic BP was a significant predictor of CV risk and was significantly better at predicting CV risk than conventionally measured systolic BP (Figure 3-2).

Comparing Clinic, Home, and Ambulatory Blood Pressure Monitoring

Not many studies have compared all three measurements of BP. However, in one recent study, a group of hypertensive patients with LVH were started on treatment with an ACE inhibitor. Patients were then followed over the subsequent months and had BPs measured using ABPM, home devices, and conventional office devices. LVH was assessed using echocardiography. The study demonstrated that there was a significantly greater correlation between LVH with BP as measured by ABPM than with BP measured by home BP monitoring. Similarly, home BP monitoring was a better predictor

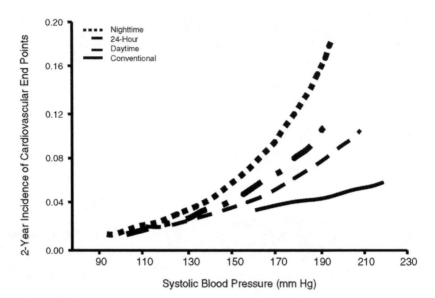

Figure 3-2 Systolic blood pressure on conventional, 24-hour, daytime, and nighttime measurement at entry as predictors of the 2-year incidence of Cardiovascular end point in the placebo group. Incidence is given as a fraction (i.e., 0.02 is an incidence of 2 events per 100 people. Using multiple Cox regression, the event rate was standardized to female sex, 69.6 years (mean age), no previous cardiovascular complications, nonsmoker status, and residence in western Europe.

of LVH regression than office BP measurement. In fact, office BP did not correlate significantly with LVH regression at all in this study.

Although ABPM is a very powerful predictor of pending CVD in hypertensive patients, it remains a fairly expensive procedure and is relatively unavailable to clinicians in clinical practice. In situations such as these, office BP and home BP assessment, or a combination of both, remain excellent alternatives.

Value of Clinic Monitoring

It is not the intention of this chapter to minimize the importance of office BP measurement as a clinical marker. It should be remembered that the vast majority of data that we have showing the association between BP and CVD is based on epidemiologic studies that have only measured office BPs. Similarly, the vast majority of data that we have demonstrating the benefits of treating hypertension is derived from outcomes studies that have only measured office BP. Thus, despite the fact that office BP is not as good at predicting pending CVD as are home and ABPM, it remains a very important and useful marker of end organ damage in hypertensive patients, particularly if BP is carefully measured with a standardized method.

However, it is relevant that all of the office-based epidemiologic data we have includes patients with white coat hypertension, who have a smaller risk of developing CVD than overt hypertensive patients; therefore, it is possible that mortality and morbidity rates for hypertensive patients have been somewhat diluted.

■ ■ ■

Key Points

- Blood pressure is a clinical marker of pending cardiovascular disease (CVD) that helps isolate patients at greater risk for cardiovascular events.

- Three techniques are available for measuring blood pressure: 1) clinic monitoring, 2) home monitoring, and 3) ambulatory measurement.

- The ausculatory method in clinic BP monitoring is still considered the gold standard; the diagnosis of hypertension is based on the average of two or more BP readings on each of two or more office visits.

- Home monitoring allows for a greater number of BP measurements and for readings to be done at different times of the day, which increases the accuracy of the BP representation.

- Like home monitoring, ambulatory blood pressure (ABPM) permits multiple measurements and enables measurements to be taken during the patient's normal activities.

- ABPM is the most accurate method of diagnosing hypertension; it is also better at assessing patient response to therapy than clinic monitoring and may therefore be instrumental in guiding and modifying treatment.

- Although ABPM is a very powerful predictor of pending CVD in hypertensive patients, it remains a fairly expensive procedure and is relatively unavailable to clinicians in clinical practice; in situations such as these, office and home BP assessment, or a combination of both, remain excellent alternatives.

- Home monitoring, when performed properly, is a better predictor of CVD than clinic monitoring. One study has shown that ABPM was better able to demonstrate left ventricular hypertrophy than home monitoring.

■ ■ ■

REFERENCES

1. **Prospective Studies Collaboration.** Age-specific relevance of usual blood pressure to vascular mortality: a meta-analysis of individual data for one million adults in 61 prospective studies. Lancet. 2002;360:1903-13.

2. **Kannel WB.** Blood pressure as a cardiovascular risk factor: prevention and treatment. JAMA. 1996;275:1571-6.

3. **Neaton JN, et al.** In: Laragh, et al, eds. Hypertension: Pathophysiology, Diagnosis, and Management. 2nd ed. New York: Raven; 1995:127-44.

4. The Seventh Report of the Joint National Committee on Prevention, Detection, Evaluation, and Treatment of High Blood Pressure: the JNC 7 Report. JAMA. 2003;289:2560-72.

5. **White WB, Berson AS, Robbins C, et al.** National standard for measurement of resting and ambulatory blood pressures with automated sphygmomanometers. Hypertension. 1993;21:504-9.

6. **O'Brien E, Petrie J, Littler W, et al.** The British Hypertension Society protocol for the evaluation of automated and semiautomated blood pressure measuring devices with special reference to ambulatory systems. J Hypertens. 1990;8:607-19.

7. **O'Brien E, Atkins N, Staessen J.** State of the market. A review of ambulatory blood pressure monitoring devices. Hypertension. 1995;26:835-42.

8. **White WB, Schulman P, McCabe EJ, Dey HM.** Average daily blood pressure, not office pressure, determines cardiac function in patients with hypertension. JAMA. 1989;261:873-7.

9. **Kuwajima I, Miyao M, Uno A, et al.** Diagnostic value of electrocardiography and echocardiography for white-coat hypertension in the elderly. Am J Cardiol. 1994;73:1232-4.

10. **Cardillo C, De Felice F, Campia U, Folli G.** Psychophysiological reactivity and cardiac end-organ changes in white-coat hypertension. Hypertension. 1993;21:836-44.

11. **Bristow JD, Honour AJ, Pickering TG, Sleight P.** Cardiovascular and respiratory changes during sleep in normal and hypertensive subjects. Cardiovasc Res. 1969;3:476-85.

12. **Millar-Craig MW, Bishop CN, Raftery EB.** Circadian variation of blood-pressure. Lancet. 1978;1:795-7.

13. **Halberg F, Halberg E, Halberg J, Halberg F.** Chronobiologic assessment of human blood pressure variation in health and disease. In: Weber MA, Drayer JIM, eds. Ambulatory Blood Pressure Monitoring. New York: Springer Verlag; 1984:137-56.

14. **Muller JE, Stone PH, Turi ZG, et al.** Circadian variation in the frequency of onset of acute myocardial infarction. N Engl J Med. 1985;313:1315-22.

15. **Thompson DR, Blandford RL, Sutton TW, Marchant PR.** Time of onset of chest pain in acute myocardial infarction. Int J Cardiol. 1985;7:139-48.

16. **Hansen O, Johansson BW, Gullberg B.** Circadian distribution of onset of acute myocardial infarction in subgroups from analysis of 10,791 patients treated in a single center. Am J Cardiol. 1992;69:1003-8.

17. **Goldberg RJ, Brady P, Muller JE, et al.** Time of onset of symptoms of acute myocardial infarction. Am J Cardiol. 1990;66:140-4.

18. **Willich SN, Levy D, Rocco MB, et al.** Circadian variation in the incidence of sudden cardiac death in the Framingham Heart Study population. Am J Cardiol. 1987;60:801-6.

19. **Shimada K, Kawamoto A, Matsubayashi K, et al.** Diurnal blood pressure variation and silent cerebrovascular damage in elderly patients with hypertension. J Hypertens. 1992;10:875-8.

20. **Kario K, Matsuo T, Kobayashi H, et al.** Nocturnal fall of blood pressure and silent cerebrovascular damage in elderly hypertensive subjects: advanced silent cerebrovascular damage in extreme dippers. Hypertension. 1996;27:130-5.

21. **Liu JE, Roman MJ, Pini R, et al.** Cardiac and arterial target organ damage in adults with elevated ambulatory and normal office blood pressure. Ann Int Med. 1999;131:564-72.

22. **Kario K, Pickering T, Umeda Y, et al.** Morning surge in blood pressure as a predictor of silent and clinical cerebrovascular disease in elderly hypertensives: a prospective study. Circulation. 2003;107:1401-6.

23. **Neutel JM, Schnaper HW, Cheung DG, et al.** Evaluation of the 24-hour blood pressure effects of beta blockers given once daily. Am J Hypertens. 1990;3: 114A.

24. **Parati G, Pomidossi G, Albini F, et al.** Relationship of 24-hour blood pressure mean and variability to severity of target-organ damage in hypertension. J Hypertens. 1987;5:93-8.

25. **Staessen JA, Thijs L, Clement D, et al.** Ambulatory blood pressure decreases on long-term placebo in older patients with isolated systolic hypertension. J Hypertens. 1994;12:1035-9.

26. **Palatini P, Mormino P, Canali C, et al.** Factors affecting ambulatory blood pressure reproducibility. Results of the HARVEST trial. Hypertension. 1994;23: 211-6.

27. **Mansoor GA, McCabe EJ, White WB.** Long-term reproducibility of ambulatory blood pressure. J Hypertens. 1994;12:703-8.

28. **Kleinert HD, Harshfield GA, Pickering TG, et al.** What is the value of home blood pressure measurement in patients with mild hypertension? Hypertension. 1984;6:574-8.

29. **Verdecchia P, Bentivoglia M, Providenza M, et al.** Reliability of home self-recorded arterial pressure in essential hypertension in relation to the stage of the disease. In: Germano G, ed. Blood Pressure Recording in the Clinical Management of Hypertension. Rome: Ediziono Pozzi; 1985:40-42.

30. **Abe H, Yokouchi M, Saitoh F, et al.** Hypertensive complications and home blood pressure: comparison with blood pressure measured in the doctor's office. J Clin Hypertens. 1987;3:661-9.

31. **Ohkubo T, Imai Y, Tsuji I, et al.** Reference values for 24-hour ambulatory blood pressure monitoring based on a prognostic criterion: the Ohasama Study. Hypertension. 1998;32:225-59.

32. **Tsuji I, Imai Y, Nagai K, et al.** Proposal of reference values for home blood pressure measurement: prognostic criteria based on a prospective observation of the general population in Ohasama, Japan. Am J Hypertens. 1997;10:409-18.

33. **Imai Y, Ohkubo T, Tsuji I, et al.** Prognostic value of ambulatory and home blood pressure measurements in comparison to screening blood pressure measurements: a pilot study in Ohasama. Blood Pressure Monit. 1996;1(Suppl 2):S51-S58.

34. **Staessen JA, Thijs L, Fagard R, et al,** for the Systolic Hypertension in Europe (Syst-Eur) Trial Investigators. Predicting cardiovascular risk using conventional vs ambulatory blood pressure in older patients with systolic hypertension. JAMA. 1999;282:539-46.

35. **Mancia G, Zanchetti A, Agabiti-Rosei E, et al.** Ambulatory blood pressure is superior to clinic blood pressure in predicting treatment-induced regression of left ventricular hypertrophy. SAMPLE Study Group. Study on Ambulatory Monitoring of Blood Pressure and Lisinopril Evaluation. Circulation. 1997;95:1464-70.

4

■ ■ ■

Principles of Hypertension
Treatment: How Low Should You Go?

Jan N. Basile, MD

Marvin Moser, MD

Elevations in blood pressure (BP) exert a strong and continuous relationship with no threshold of risk for developing cardiovascular disease. Both systolic BP (SBP) and diastolic BP (DBP) are independently related to cardiovascular risk (1). For persons aged 40 to 70 years, the risk of cardiovascular disease begins at 115/75 mm Hg and doubles with each 20/10 mm Hg incremental increase up to 185/115 mm Hg (2). For persons 50 years of age and older, an SBP elevation is a more important risk factor for cardiovascular disease than an elevation in DBP (3,4). Currently, there are essentially two targets for BP control: <140/90 mm Hg for individuals without evidence of diabetes or renal disease, and <130/80 mm Hg for patients with these diseases. Many persons with hypertension will require two or more antihypertensive medications to achieve BP control. When reducing SBP to a goal of <140 mm Hg, caution should be exercised if DBP is lowered to <55 mm Hg.

Currently Recommended Blood Pressure Targets

More people today are aware of and are on therapy for hypertension than in previous years, but control rates, which are improving, are still achieved in only one in three people (4). Since the late 1970s, the minimum goal for BP reduction for most patients with hypertension has been <140/90 mm Hg. The National Heart Lung and Blood Institute has issued several reports on high BP. In its Seventh Report on the Prevention, Detection, Evaluation, and Treatment of High Blood Pressure (JNC-7), the panel recommended an

Table 4-1   Blood Pressure Treatment Goals

- <140 mm Hg for patients without diabetes or evidence of coronary heart disease

- <130/80 mm Hg for patients with diabetes or coronary heart disease

* As recommended by the JNC-7 Report.

even lower goal for higher-risk patients (including diabetics and those with renal impairment) to <130/80 mm Hg (Table 4-1). Whereas the JNC VI in 1997 recommended a target BP of <125/75 mm Hg for patients with renal impairment and more than a gram per day of urinary protein, this goal, discussed below, is no longer recommended (5).

Clinical Benefits of Achieving Blood Pressure Targets

Clinical trials over the past 35 years have proven the benefits of antihypertensive therapy in reducing the rates of stroke, heart failure, and heart attack. It is of interest to examine the benefits in trials where attempts were made to reach targets similar to those listed above. The first placebo-controlled cooperative hypertension trial, which targeted DBP reductions, was conducted in 1967 by the Veterans Administration (VA) (6). Performed in 143 US veterans with severe hypertension (supine DBP 115-129 mm Hg), the study was stopped prematurely without any statistical analysis because there was a major improvement in prognosis on active therapy. There were no deaths in patients on active therapy compared with four deaths on placebo with one hospitalization on active therapy and 27 for those on placebo when BP was reduced to <105 mm Hg. A follow-up study also under the direction of the VA showed that lowering DBP to <90 mm Hg further improved cardiovascular outcome. Several subsequent large, prospective placebo-controlled hypertension trials conducted in the 1970s, 1980s, and 1990s found a reduction in cardiovascular morbidity and mortality in treated compared with control patients (Table 4-2). These have been summarized in several recent meta-analyses, which show a 38% reduction in stroke, 16% reduction in heart attack, 52% reduction in heart failure, 21% reduction in cardiovascular death, and a 35% reduction in left ventricular hypertrophy in treated compared with placebo or control subjects (7-11).

There is no longer any doubt that controlling BP reduces cardiovascular complications from hypertension. The minimum goal set for BP reduction has been SBP <140 mm Hg and DBP <90 mm Hg. In the controlled clinical trials, more than 20%-30% of patients did not achieve these goal BPs. Despite this fact, cardiovascular events were significantly reduced. In more recent trials, a higher percentage of patients receiving treatment have achieved goal BPs. About 90% of hypertensive patients have had their DBP reduced to <90 mm Hg in the Hypertension Optimal Treatment (HOT), the

Table 4-2 Effects of Therapy in Older Hypertensive Patients

	Clinical Trial							
	Australian	EWPHE	C & W	STOP	MRC	SHEP	HDFP	Syst Eur
Number of patients	582	840	884	1,627	4,396	4,736	2,374	4,695
Age range (years)	60-69	>60	60-79	70-84	64-74	60-80	60-69	>60
Mean BP at entry (mm Hg)	165/101	182/101	197/100	195/102	185/91	170/77	170/101	174/86

Percent Reduction of Events in Treated Compared with Control Patients

	Australian	EWPHE	C & W	STOP	MRC	SHEP	HDFP	Syst Eur
Stroke	33	36	42*	47*	25*	33*	44*	42*
CAD	18	20	+0.03	13†	19	27*	15*	30
CHF	—	22	32	51*	—	55*	—	29
All CVD	31	29*	24*	40*	17*	32*	16*	31*

EWPHE, European Working Party on High Blood Pressure in the Elderly; C & W, Coope and Warrender; STOP, Swedish Trial in Older Patients with Hypertension; MRC, Medical Research Council Study; SHEP, Systolic Hypertension in the Elderly Program; HDFP, Hypertension Detection and Follow-up Program; Syst Eur, Systolic Hypertension in Europe Multicentre Trial; CAD, coronary artery disease; CHF, congestive heart failure; CVD, cerebrovascular disease.

* Statistically significant.

† Myocardial infarction only; sudden deaths decreased from 13 to 4.

Republished with permission from Moser M. Clinical Management of Hypertension. 6th ed. Caddo, OK: Professional Communications; 2002.

Antihypertensive and Lipid-Lowering Treatment to Prevent Heart Attack Trial (ALLHAT), and the Controlled Onset Verapamil Investigation of Cardiovascular Endpoints (CONVINCE) trials; only about 60% of subjects had SBPs reduced to <140 mm Hg (12-14).

Benefits of Treating Isolated Systolic Hypertension

While the observed risk of an elevated SBP on cardiovascular disease has been known for over 40 years, specific recommendations for treating isolated systolic hypertension (ISH) were first published in the JNC V report in 1993 (15). Well-designed, randomized, placebo-controlled trials have shown benefit from drug treatment in elderly patients with ISH. In those patients with stage 2 ISH (SBP >160 mm Hg and DBP <90-95 mm Hg), a reduction in stroke, heart failure, coronary events, and mortality was found. Benefit occurred when SBP was reduced by at least 20 mm Hg below the entry SBP, to either 150 or 160 mm Hg (16,17). In many patients benefit was noted despite the fact that BPs <140 mm Hg were not achieved.

A recent meta-analysis of eight placebo-controlled trials included 15,693 patients 60 years of age and older with ISH. It reported that active treatment over a 3.8-year period of time reduced coronary events by 23%, stroke by 30%, cardiovascular death by 18%, and overall mortality by 13% (18). In patients older than 70 years of age, the absolute benefit was even greater. Treating 19 patients for 5 years prevented one major fatal or nonfatal cardiovascular event. Most trials involve patients 60 to 80 years of age, but there are many in the over-80 age group: a recent meta-analysis supports the benefit of antihypertensive therapy in patients over 80 years of age (Table 4-3) (19). While a diuretic and a calcium-channel blocker are the only drugs that have been specifically tested as initial therapy against a placebo in elderly patients with ISH (now defined as a BP >140/<90-95 mm Hg but defined in these trials as >160/<90 mm Hg), additional therapy was required in up to 50% of patients (16-17). In several comparative, non-placebo-controlled trials, which included many patients with ISH, use of an ACE-I or a beta-blocker-based regimen often with a diuretic, resulted in a decrease in BP. Although it is not always possible to achieve goal BP in all patients, a high percentage of patients with ISH were successfully treated, achieving SBP <140 mm Hg in the controlled trials.

Benefit of Reducing Blood Pressure to <140 mm Hg in the ISH Patient

Is there clinical trial evidence to recommend a goal SBP <140 mm Hg in patients with ISH? Only a few clinical trials have specifically attempted to randomize patients to different target levels of BP as a primary intervention,

Table 4-3   Results of Antihypertensive Drug Therapy in Patients >80 Years of Age*

• *Significant reduction of:* ➤ >35% in strokes (mostly nonfatal) ➤ >35% in heart failure ➤ >20% in cardiovascular events	• Nonsignificant reduction of about 20% in major coronary events • Nonsignificant increase of about 10% to 15% in total mortality

* Based on results in >1800 patients.
Republished with permission from Gueyffier F, Bulpitt C, Goissel JP, et al. Antihypertensive drugs in very old people: a subgroup meta-analysis of randomized controlled trials. INDANA Group. Lancet. 1999;353:793-96.

and no specific trial has targeted BP <140 mm Hg in those with ISH. Many recommendations on the benefits of achieving SBP <140 mm Hg come from epidemiologic observation or post hoc analyses of clinical trial data. One such post hoc analysis was published almost 10 years after the original results of the SHEP trial (20). In this analysis, performed on the original 4736 subjects 60 years of age or older with SBP >160 mm Hg and DBP <90 mm Hg, the risk of stroke was calculated according to on-treatment BP during follow-up. Those that achieved the original goal of the trial, SBP <160 mm Hg and at least a 20 mm Hg reduction from baseline, had a 33% reduction in stroke. The patients who achieved SBP <150 mm Hg did even better, with a 38% risk reduction in stroke. The group who achieved SBP <140 mm Hg had a 22% reduction in stroke risk, which did not reach statistical significance because of the smaller numbers of patients involved. These data should not be interpreted to mean that achieving SBP <140 mm Hg is less beneficial than achieving a higher SBP level. They do suggest, however, that if SBP is reduced at least 20 mm Hg from baseline, even if not to the presently recommended goal of <140 mm Hg, clinical outcome is still improved.

Although the vascular risk of stage 1 ISH (SBP 140 to 159 mm Hg and DBP <90 mm Hg) is well established, no treatment trial has been completed to test whether an improvement in outcome occurs in these individuals if BP is lowered to a specific goal. Several trials in patients with stage 1 ISH that affects 25% of the elderly population are ongoing.

While none of the clinical trials in patients with ISH achieved SBP <140 mm Hg, JNC 7 and a recent consensus statement from the National High BP Education Program have recommended a decrease in SBP to <140 mm Hg in patients with ISH (4,21).

Cardiovascular and Renal Benefits of Reducing Blood Pressure to Lower Than 130/80 mm Hg in Diabetic Patients

Diabetics are most likely to die of atherosclerotic vascular disease, the risk of which is accelerated by hypertension. The risk of stroke or any cardiovascular event is almost doubled in hypertensive patients with diabetes mellitus. In addition, diabetes is the number one cause of end-stage renal disease. There exists a nearly linear relationship between elevations in BP and the rate of decline in kidney function. Current recommendations state that BP should be reduced in diabetics to <130/80 (4). Is there sufficient evidence to justify this recommendation?

The United Kingdom Prospective Diabetes Study (UKPDS) was performed in 1148 type 2 diabetics (22). It involved simultaneous randomizations to study both the effects of different initial antihypertensive medications (a treatment regimen comparing the ACE inhibitor captopril to the beta-blocker atenolol), as well as two different BP goals (BP target of 150/85 mm Hg compared to a target of <180/105 mm Hg). There was no difference in outcome between the captopril- and atenolol-based treatment groups after an average 8.4-year follow-up. The 758 patients randomized to the "tight" BP goal of <150/85 mm Hg (who achieved an average BP of 144/82 mm Hg) experienced fewer cardiovascular events than the 390 randomized to the "less tight" goal of <180/105 mm Hg (who achieved an average BP of 154/87 mm Hg). Participants in the lower BP group had a risk reduction of 32% in diabetes-related deaths, 24% reduction in diabetes-related endpoints (including amputations), 44% reduction in strokes, and 37% reduction in microvascular complications (including nephropathy and advanced retinopathy requiring photocoagulation) (Table 4-4). Thus, a BP difference of only -10/-5 mm Hg resulted in a significant risk reduction in diabetes-related cardiovascular and micro-vascular (including renal) complications. While the achieved BP difference between the two groups support the clinical benefit

---

Table 4-4   Comparative Study of ACE Inhibitor and β-Blocker Treatment Programs in UKPDS*

- Number of patients in study (non–insulin-dependent diabetics): 1148

- Tight blood pressure control: achieved blood pressure of 144/82 mm Hg compared with group with blood pressure of 154/87 mm Hg

- Reduction in cardiovascular risk—tight: less effective blood pressure control

- Reduction in events:
  - ➤ Strokes   44%
  - ➤ Heart failure   56%
  - ➤ Deaths related to diabetes   32%
  - ➤ Microvascular disease   37%
  - ➤ Myocardial infarction and sudden death (not significant)   21%

- No difference in outcome between different treatment groups; difference in achieved blood pressure accounted for difference in outcome

UKPDS = United Kingdom Prospective Diabetes Study. Republished with permission from Turner R, Holman R, Stratton I, et al., for the United Kingdom Prospective Diabetes Study Group. Tight blood pressure control and risk of macrovascular and microvascular complications in type 2 diabetes: UKPDS 38. BMJ. 1998;317:707-713.

associated with a lower-than-usual BP for the diabetic hypertensive, the achieved BPs were still above the recommended goal of <130/80 mm Hg.

A post hoc analysis of the UKPDS found that for each 10 mm Hg reduction in SBP, additional risk reductions occurred in both macrovascular (atherosclerotic) and microvascular events: 15% for death related to diabetes, 11% for myocardial infarction, 12% for any complication related to diabetes, and 13% for microvascular complications (23). In this analysis, no threshold for lowering BP was observed, with the lowest risk of complications found in diabetics whose SBP was <120 mm Hg. The authors concluded that while any reduction in SBP reduces the risk of complications from diabetes, the greater the reduction in BP the better.

Additional data on benefit from a reduction in SBP on cardiovascular outcome were also reported in a post hoc analyses of the diabetic cohorts within the SHEP and Systolic Hypertension in Europe (Syst-Eur) trials (24,25). Diabetics with SBP <140 mm Hg had a greater cardiovascular disease risk reduction when compared with those with higher BP levels, whereas those who could achieve levels <130 mm Hg had an even greater reduction in cardiovascular disease risk (24,25).

In addition to a reduction in risk, post hoc analyses of several clinical trials have noted an improvement in renal outcome when SBP was lowered to <140 mm Hg. Although clinical trial evidence supports reducing SBP to <130 mm Hg in Type 1 diabetics with evidence of nephropathy, no prospective clinical trial has evaluated the same target in Type 2 diabetics (26). The current recommendation for reducing SBP to <130 mm Hg in all diabetics comes from post hoc and observational analysis (27).

The Appropriate Blood Pressure Control in Diabetes trial randomized Type 2 diabetic subjects with hypertension to different levels of BP control in an attempt to determine how low to go and whether lowering BP makes a difference in outcome. This study showed no difference in decline of renal function based on BP level achieved over a 5-year follow-up period (28). It should be noted, however, in the normotensive cohort of this same trial, that the progression to incipient and overt nephropathy, progression to retinopathy, and the risk of stroke were all diminished in those who maintained SBP <130 mm Hg (actually achieved 128/75 mm Hg) (29).

The degree of reduction in DBP on benefit was also tested in the Hypertension Optimal Treatment trial (12). Of the 18,790 patients in the overall clinical trial, a diabetic sub-study evaluated 1501 type 2 diabetic patients who were randomized to one of three DBP goals: ≤90, ≤85, or ≤80 mm Hg. After 3.8 years of follow-up, patients randomized to ≤80 mm Hg had a 51% reduction in the total risk of heart attack, stroke, or death, the primary endpoint, compared with those whose DBP was ≤90 mm Hg (Table 4-5). Mean achieved BPs in the two groups were 81 and 85 mm Hg, respectively. Even when other endpoints were compared (e.g., including "silent" myocardial infarction or cardiovascular death), the group randomized to the lowest DBP had the best prognosis. While the average achieved

---

Table 4-5   Summary of the Hypertension Optimal Treatment (HOT) Trial

- No significant difference in cardiovascular (CV) events or total mortality in subjects with achieved target diastolic blood pressures (DBPs) of 85, 83, or 81 mm Hg
- Most of the benefit achieved with BPs of −140/85-90 mm Hg
- Overall event rate lower than in previous studies, probably because of pronounced lowering of BP (only 8.5% of subjects ended with DBPs >90 mm Hg compared with about 20% to 30% in previous trials)
- In patients with diabetes mellitus:
  - ➤ Major CV events and mortality reduced significantly greater in target group (<80 mm Hg compared to <90 mm Hg)
  - ➤ No significant difference in strokes, all myocardial infarctions (MIs), or total mortality
- In patients with ischemic heart disease: no significant difference in major CV events between target groups with DBPs <90, <85, and <80 mm Hg

Republished with permission from Hansson L, Zanchetti A, Carruthers SG, et al: Effects of intensive blood-pressure lowering and low-dose aspirin in patients with hypertension: principal results of the Hypertension Optimal Treatment (HOT) randomized trial. HOT Study Group. Lancet 351:1755-1762, 1998.

SBP in this trial was 138 mm Hg, lower trends in cardiovascular events were noted for those whose SBP was <130 mm Hg.

In summary, epidemiologic data indicate that BPs of 120/70 mm Hg or above are associated with an increase in cardiovascular morbidity and mortality in persons with diabetes. The recommendation to lower BP in the diabetic patient to 130/80 mm Hg is at present evidence-based only for DBP. While no clinical trial has specifically tested the renal benefits for achieving the currently recommended SBP goal of <130 mm Hg in the diabetic, observational studies in both the diabetic and nondiabetic demonstrate that SBP levels between 130 and 135 mm Hg markedly improve kidney disease outcome compared with levels above 140 mm Hg (27,30). Based on these findings, the American Diabetes Association, the National Kidney Foundation, the British Hypertension Society, and the JNC 7 all recommend a BP of <130/80 mm Hg in diabetic patients to reduce cardiovascular morbidity and mortality and to maximally preserve renal function (4,27,31,32). Whether achieving lower levels of SBP will reduce cardiovascular risk is being evaluated in the Action to Control Cardiovascular Risk in Diabetes trial, in which SBP 120 mm Hg is being compared with SBP 140 mm Hg. The results will not be known for several years.

Benefits of Reducing Blood Pressure to <130/80 mm Hg in Patients with Renal Disease

The Sixth JNC report recommended BP <125/75 mm Hg for patients with more than one gram of proteinuria per day (33). This was based on a post hoc analysis of the "Modification of Diet in Renal Disease" study whose primary purpose was to see if a lower intake of dietary protein would have a beneficial effect on the progression of renal impairment. All 585 subjects with chronic renal insufficiency were randomized to both different levels of dietary protein intake and different BP targets (mean arterial pressure [MAP] <107 mm Hg or <92 mm Hg, corresponding to cuff BPs of <140/90 mm Hg or 125/75 mm Hg). There were no significant differences in progression of renal disease, hospitalization, or death between randomized groups for either intervention (34). Since the achieved MAP in the two randomized groups turned out to be only slightly different (93.0±7.3 vs. 97.7±7.7 mm Hg), both BP groups were pooled and stratified according to level of baseline proteinuria. For every 1 mm Hg increase in MAP there was a 35% increase in the risk of hospitalization for cardiovascular disease (35). Based on this post hoc analysis, JNC VI recommended a target BP of <125/75 mm Hg for patients with more than one gram per day of proteinuria.

More recently, the African American Study on Kidney Disease (AASK) was conducted in non-diabetic patients with renal disease and hypertension (36). Individuals were randomized to one of three antihypertensive agents and one of two BP goals. African Americans with proteinuria randomized to the calcium antagonist amlodipine experienced more renal disease progression than those randomized to the ACE inhibitor ramipril. Of interest, those randomized to the MAP of <92 mm Hg (corresponding to BP <125/75 mm Hg) had no further improvement in renal function compared to those randomized to the higher MAP between 102 and 107 mm Hg (corresponding to BP 140/90 mm Hg). Most individuals, however, did not have more than 1 gram of proteinuria at baseline. Based mostly on the AASK results published since JNC VI, recommendations have changed; it is no longer recommended that BP be reduced to <125/75 mm Hg in patients with renal disease and significant proteinuria. The recommended targeted BP to protect against cardiovascular disease and nephropathy in diabetics and non-diabetics with underlying renal disease is now <130/80 mm Hg. This is based on reasonably good scientific evidence.

Are There Any Dangers of Excessive Blood Pressure Lowering?

While the lowering of elevated BP can lead to an improvement in cardiovascular outcome, some studies have observed an increase in cardiovascular events when BP was reduced below a critical value (of about 80-85 mm Hg). This "J-shaped curve" effect hypothesizes that lowering DBP below a certain value in individuals with underlying cardiovascular disease increases the risk of cardiovascular death. The HOT study was designed to test this question. This trial was prospective, randomized, and open with blinded end-point and assigned 18,790 hypertensive patients from 26 countries (mean age, 61.5 years) to a target DBP <80 mm Hg, <85 mm Hg, or <90 mm Hg. After an average 3.8 years of follow-up, only a small 2 mm Hg difference (less than the expected 5 mm Hg difference) was achieved among the three groups (85, 83, and 81 mm Hg). While no benefit was seen in the non-diabetic group that achieved the lowest DBP, no increase in cardiovascular events occurred either (achieved DBP 81 mm Hg versus achieved 85 mm Hg). The "optimum" BP to prevent cardiovascular events was 138.5/82.6 mm Hg (12).

While the HOT study found no evidence of a "J-curve effect," a retrospective analysis of the SHEP trial recently found that in the few patients whose DBP was lowered to <55 mm Hg, no benefit in outcome occurred when compared with those in the placebo group. Thus, until further prospective trials examine this question, it appears prudent to exercise caution if DBP decreases to <55 mm Hg in older individuals with ISH (37). As noted elsewhere, this is an unusual occurrence (38).

Conclusions

Reducing blood pressure to as close to established goal levels as possible is associated with less cardiovascular and renal disease than if BP remains uncontrolled. Despite the fact that many patients who experienced benefit in the clinical trials did not achieve ideal BP levels, there is enough evidence to recommend that in patients with uncomplicated hypertension a reasonable goal should be <140/90 mm Hg. In diabetics or patients with renal impairment a lower goal of <130/80 mm Hg is recommended. Currently, only 34% of hypertensive Americans are treated to goal BPs.

■   ■   ■

Key Points

- Although current guidelines suggest the minimum goal for BP reduction is SBP <140 mm Hg and DBP <90 mm Hg, there is more evidence for the DBP goal than the SBP goal.

- The current guidleines suggest SBP be lowered to <140 mm Hg in those with ISH, but clinical trial evidence suggests benefit occurs when SBP is reduced by at least 20 mm Hg below the entry SBP, to either 150 or 160 mm Hg.

- Epidemiologic observation shows that BPs of 120/70 mm Hg or below are associated with the least cardiovascular morbidity and mortality in those with diabetes; however, the recommendation to lower BP in diabetic patients to <130/80 mm Hg is evidence-based for DBP only. The ACCORD trial is evaluating the ideal SBP goal.

- Based mostly on the AASK trial, the current goal for BP reduction in both diabetics and non-diabetics to protect against cardiovascular disease and nephropathy in those with underlying renal disease should be <130/80 mm Hg.

- Until further prospective trials examine the question, it appears prudent to exercise caution when lowering DBP to <55 mm Hg in older individuals with ISH.

■   ■   ■

REFERENCES

1. **Kannel WB.** Elevated SBP as a cardiovascular risk factor. Am J Cardiol. 2000;15:251-5.

2. **Lewington S, Clarke R, Qizilbash N, et al.** Age-specific relevance of usual BP to vascular mortality. Lancet. 2002;360:1903-13.

3. **Kannel WB, Schwartz MJ, McNamara PM.** BP and risk of coronary heart disease. The Framingham Study. Dis Chest. 1969;56:43-62.

4. The Seventh Report of the Joint National Committee on Prevention, Detection, Evaluation, and Treatment of High BP The JNC 7 Report. JAMA. 2003;289:2560-72.

5. The Sixth Report of the Joint National Committee on Prevention, Detection, Evaluation, and Treatment of High BP (JNC VI). Arch Intern Med. 1997;157:2413-46.

6. Veterans Administration Cooperative Study Group on Antihypertensive Agents. Effects of treatment on morbidity in hypertension: results in patients with DBP averaging 115 through 129 mm Hg. JAMA. 1967;202:1028-34.

7. **Moser M, Hebert PR.** Prevention of disease progression, left ventricular hypertrophy and congestive heart failure in hypertension treatment trials. J Am Coll Cardiol. 1996;27:1214-8.

8. **Psaty BM, Smith NL, Siscovick DS, et al.** Health outcomes associated with antihypertensive therapies used as first-line agents: a systematic review and meta-analysis. JAMA. 1997;277:739-45.

9. BP Lowering Treatment Trialists' Collaborative. Effects of ACE-inhibitors, calcium antagonists, and other blood-pressure-lowering drugs: Results of prospectively designed overviews of randomised trials. Lancet. 2000;356:1955-64.

10. **Hebert PR, Moser M, Mayer J, Hennekens CH.** Recent evidence on drug therapy of mild to moderate hypertension and decreased risk of coronary heart disease. Arch Intern Med. 1993;153:578-81.

11. **Lloyd-Jones DM, Evans JC, Larson MG, et al.** Differential control of systolic and DBP. Factors asssociated with lack of BP control in the community. Hypertension. 2000; 36:504-9.

12. **Hansson L, Zanchetti A, Carruthers SG, et al.** Effects of intensive blood-pressure lowering and low-dose aspirin in patients with hypertension: principal results of the Hypertension Optimal Treatment (HOT) randomized trial. HOT Study Group. Lancet. 1998;351:1755-62.

13. Major outcomes in high-risk hypertensive patients randomized to angiotensin-converting enzyme inhibitor or calcium channel blocker vs diuretic. The Antihypertensive and Lipid-Lowering Treatment to Prevent Heart Attack Trial (ALLHAT). JAMA. 2002;288:2981-97.

14. **Black HR, Elliot WJ, Grandist G, et al. for the CONVINCE Research Group.** Principal results of the Controlled Onset Verapamil Investigation of Cardiovascular Endpoints (CONVINCE) trial. JAMA. 2003;289:2073-82.

15. The Fifth Report of the Joint National Committee on Prevention, Detection, Evaluation, and Treatment of High BP (JNC V). Arch Intern Med. 1993;153:154-83.

16. **SHEP Cooperative Research Group.** Prevention of stroke by antihypertensive drug treatment in older persons with isolated systolic hypertension. JAMA. 1991; 265: 3255-64.

17. **Staessen JA, Fagard R, Thijs L, et al.** Morbidity and mortality in the placebo controlled European trial on isolated systolic hypertension (Syst-Eur) in the elderly. Lancet. 1997;350:757-64.

18. **Staessen JA, Gasowski J, Wang JC, et al.** Risk of untreated and treated isolated systolic hypertension in the elderly: Meta-analysis of outcome trials. Lancet. 2000;355:865-72.

19. **Gueyffier F, Bulpitt C, Goissel JP, et al.** Antihypertensive drugs in very old people: a subgroup metanalysis of randomized controlled trials. INDANA Group. Lancet. 1999;353:793-6.

20. **Perry HM Jr, Davis BR, Price TR, et al.** Effect of treating isolated systolic hypertension on the risk of developing various types and subtypes of stroke. The Systolic Hypertension in the Elderly Program (SHEP). JAMA. 2000;284:465-71.

21. **Izzo J, Levy D, Black HR.** Clinical Advisory Statement. Importance of SBP in older Americans. Hypertension. 2000;35:1021-4.

22. **Turner R, Holman R, Stratton I, et al for the United Kingdom Prospective Diabetes Study Group.** Tight BP control and risk of macrovascular and microvascular complications in type 2 diabetes: UKPDS 38. BMJ. 1998;317:707-13.

23. **Adler AI, Stratton IM, Neil HA, et al.** Association of SBP with macrovascular or microvascular complications of type 2 diabetes: UKPDS 36. BMJ. 2000;312: 412-9.

24. **Curb JD, Pressel SL, Cutler JA, et al.** Effect of diuretic-based antihypertensive treatment on cardiovascular disease risk in older diabetic patients with isolated systolic hypertension. Systolic Hypertension in the Elderly Program Cooperative Research Group. JAMA. 1996;276:1886-92.

25. **Tuomilehto J, Rastenyte D, Birkenhager WH, et al.** Effects of calcium-channel blockade in older patients with diabetes and systolic hypertension. Systolic Hypertension in Europe Trial Investigators. N Engl J Med 1999;340:677-84.

26. **Lewis JB, Berl T, Bain RP, et al.** Effect of intensive BP control on the course of type 1 diabetic nephropathy. Collaborative Study Group. Am J Kidney Dis. 1999; 34:809-17.

27. **Bakris GL, Williams M, Dworkin L, et al.** Preserving renal function in adults with hypertension and diabetes: a consensus approach. National Kidney Foundation Hypertension and Diabetes Executive Committees Working Group. Am J Kidney Dis. 2000;36:646-61.

28. **Estacio RO, Jeffers BW, Gifford N, Schrier RW.** Effect of BP control on diabetic microvascular complications in patients with hypertension and type 2 diabetes. Diabetes Care. 2000;Suppl 2:B54-B64.

29. **Schrier RW, Estacio RO, Esler A, Mehler P.** Effects of aggressive BP control in normotensive type 2 diabetic patients on albuminuria, retinopathy and strokes. Kidney Int. 2002:61:1086-97.

30. **Ravid M, Lang R, Rachmani R, Lishner M.** Long-term renoprotective effect of angiotensin-convertine enzyme inhibition in non-insulin-dependent diabetes mellitus. A 7-year follow-up study. Arch Intern Med. 1996;156:286-9.

31. American Diabetes Association: clinical practice recommendations 2002. Diabetes Care. 2002;25(Suppl 1):S1-147.

32. **Ramsay LE, Williams B, Johnston GD, et al.** British Hypertension Society Guidelines for hypertension management 1999: Summary. BMJ. 1999;319:630-5.

33. The Sixth report of the Joint National Committee on Prevention, Detection, Evaluation, and Treatment of High BP (JNC VI). Arch Intern Med. 1997;157:2413-46.

34. **Klahr S, Levey AS, Beck GJ, et al.** The effects of dietary protein restriction and blood-pressure control on the progression of chronic renal disease: Modification of Diet in Renal Disease Study Group. N Engl J Med. 1994;330:877-84.

35. **Lazarus JM, Bourgoignie JJ, Buckalew VM, et al for the Modification of Diet in Renal Disease Study Group.** Achievement and safety of a low BP goal in chronic renal disease: Modification of Diet in Renal Disease Study Group. Hypertension. 1997;29:641-50.

36. **Wright JT Jr, Bakris G, Greene T, et al.** African American Study of Kidney Disease and Hypertension (AASK) Study Group. Effect of BP lowering and antihypertensive drug class on progression of hypertensive kidney disease. JAMA. 2002;288:2421-31.

37. **Somes G, Pahor M, Shorr RI, et al.** The role of DBP when treating isolated systolic hypertension. Arch Intern Med. 1999;159:2004-9.

38. **Moser M.** Clinical Management of Hypertension. 6th ed. Caddo, OK: Professional Communications, 2002.

5

■ ■ ■

Nonpharmacological Therapy of Hypertension

Connie Mere, MD
Vasilios Papademetriou, MD

The JNC in its Seventh Report recommends adoption of healthy lifestyles by all persons for the prevention and management of hypertension. Lifestyle modifications may also be useful in patients whose hypertension is being treated with pharmacologic therapy. Lifestyle modifications reduces blood pressure (BP), enhances antihypertensive drug efficacy, and decreases cardiovascular risk (1). Major lifestyle modifications shown to lower BP include weight reduction in individuals who are overweight or obese, adoption of a low-fat vegetarian-like diet (5), dietary sodium reduction, physical activity, and moderation of alcohol consumption. A 1600-mg sodium Dietary Approaches to Stop Hypertension (DASH) eating plan has been shown to have effects similar to single-drug therapy. Combinations of two or more lifestyle modifications can achieve even better results (1).

In hypertensive persons, lifestyle changes can serve as initial treatment before the start of drug therapy. They may also serve as an adjunct to medication in those who are already on drug therapy. Finally, lifestyle modifications may be used to facilitate drug step-down or drug withdrawal in highly motivated persons. In non-hypertensive persons, lifestyle changes can prevent hypertension and thus lower cardiovascular risk, especially in salt-sensitive individuals. These changes may be difficult to achieve and maintain, but emphasis should be placed on developing and implementing such strategies and interventions.

Reduced Dietary Sodium

Several studies in laboratory animals and humans show a relationship between high BP and dietary sodium (3). The International Study of Salt and Blood Pressure (INTERSALT Study), a cross-sectional study involving more than 10,000 individuals, aged 20 to 59 years in 52 population samples from 32 countries, demonstrated that 24-hour sodium excretion was significantly related to BP level, age, and prevalence of hypertension (9). In both normotensive and hypertensive subgroups, there was a lower systolic BP of 3 to 6 mm Hg per 100 mmol/d lower level of sodium excretion.

Normotensive or hypertensive persons whose BPs rise in response to high-salt diets or fall with salt restriction are termed salt-sensitive. Clinical predictors of salt sensitivity include older age, low-renin hypertension (including blacks), insulin resistance/diabetes, renal failure, and increased sympathetic activity.

Evidence of Efficacy

Several large, long-term, randomized clinical trials have shown that even a moderate reduction in sodium intake reduces BP levels. Typical sodium consumption in the United States is 150 mmol/d, whereas the upper limit of the current national recommendation is 100 mmol/d. The Trials of Hypertension Prevention, Phase II, evaluated the benefits of weight reduction and sodium reduction to achieve a target intake of 80 mmol/d, alone and in combination (6). The study participants included 2382 men and women aged 30-54 years who were slightly to moderately overweight and had normal BPs. Counseling aimed at helping participants achieve a desirable weight or more weight reduction (in the weight loss and combined groups), and sodium intake of 80 mmol/d (in the sodium reduction and combined groups) was provided. Follow-up was for 3-4 years. Sodium excretion decreased 50 and 40 mmol/d at 6 and 36 months, respectively, in the low-sodium group and resulted in BP decrease of 2.9/1.6 mm Hg compared with the usual care group. Compared with the usual care group, weight loss and reduction in sodium intake, individually and in combination, were effective at lowering systolic and diastolic BP. Maximal effects were observed in the short-term (6 months) and declined over time.

Similar benefits were demonstrated in The Trial of Nonpharmacologic Interventions in the Elderly (TONE) (7). Individuals whose BPs were controlled with 1 antihypertensive agent were enrolled in the study. The effects of weight loss and dietary salt reduction were studied. Compared with usual care group, the mean sodium reduction was 40 mmol/d. About half of the group that lost weight and reduced salt intake and one third of those who either lost weight or reduced salt intake were able to stop and remain off medication.

The DASH-Sodium Trial examined the beneficial effects of different levels of dietary sodium (50 mmol/d, 100 mmol/d, and 150 mmol/d at 2100 kcal) in conjunction with the DASH diet in persons with and without hypertension. The study was a multi-center, randomized trial comparing the effects of BP of three levels of sodium intake in two diets in adults aged 22 years and older whose average systolic BP was 120-159 mm Hg and average diastolic BP was 80-95 mm Hg on screening. Other exclusion criteria were heart disease, renal insufficiency, poorly controlled hyperlipidemia or diabetes mellitus, insulin requiring diabetes, special dietary requirements, and intake of more than 14 alcoholic drinks per week. The trial was conducted from September 1997 to November 1999. A total of 412 participants (56%-57% blacks and 54%-59% women) were randomly assigned to either a control diet (typical of what many people in the United States eat) or the DASH diet, which emphasizes fruits; vegetables; low-fat foods; whole grains; poultry; fish; nuts; and smaller amounts of red meat, sweets, and sugar-containing beverages than the typical diet in the United States.

The DASH diet also contained smaller amounts of cholesterol, total and saturated fat, and larger amounts of potassium, calcium, magnesium, dietary fiber, and protein than the typical diet. In addition, participants in both the control diet group and the DASH diet group were assigned to have their sodium intake at one of three levels: high (a target of 150 mmol/day with energy intake of 2100 kcal), intermediate (a target of 100 mmol per day), and low (a target of 50 mmol per day, reflecting the level that the investigators hypothesized might produce an additional lowering of BP.

Reducing sodium intake from the high to the intermediate level reduced the systolic BP by 2.1 mm Hg during the control diet and by 1.3 mm Hg during the DASH diet. Reducing the sodium intake from the intermediate to the low level caused additional reductions of 4.6 mm Hg during the control diet and 1.7 mm Hg during the DASH diet. The effects of sodium were observed in participants with and without hypertension, in blacks and other races, and in women and men. The DASH diet was associated with a significantly lower systolic BP at each sodium level, and the difference was greater with high sodium levels than with low levels. Compared with the control diet with a high sodium level, the DASH diet with a low sodium level led to a mean systolic BP that was 7.1 mm Hg lower in participants without hypertension and 11.5 mm Hg lower in participants with hypertension, with the greatest reduction in black hypertensive persons (11).

In a subgroup analysis of the DASH sodium diet, among non-hypertensive participants who received the control diet lower sodium intake decreased BP by 7.0/3.8 mm Hg in those older than 45 years of age and by 3.7/1.5 mm Hg in those 45 years of age or younger (12). Although several studies have shown that restricting sodium intake in people with hypertension reduces their BP, it is unclear what effects a low-sodium diet has on cardiovascular events and mortality. The Worksite Cohort Study, the National Health and Nutrition Examination Survey (NHANES) I and II Follow-up Studies, and the Multiple Risk Factor Intervention Trial (MRFIT) Follow-up Study either showed an inverse relationship or no association between estimated sodium excretion and cardiovascular events (10-13). However, there were confounders and flaws in analyses and conclusions of these studies.

Recommendations for Clinical Practice

Current guidelines recommend reducing daily dietary sodium intake to no more than 100 mmol (equivalent to 2.4 g of sodium or 6 g of sodium chloride). Approximate systolic BP reduction with this intervention is 2-8 mm Hg (16). A policy of reduction in salt intake for the entire population through reduction in salt concentrations in processed foods can achieve small reductions in BP across the whole population for sustained periods of time. Only 10% of dietary sodium comes from salt added to food at the table, so patients should be cautioned about the sodium content in processed foods. More significant reduction in BP may be achieved in a person with salt-sensitive phenotype (African-American, older age, obese, insulin-resistant diabetes mellitus, chronic kidney disease, positive family history of hypertension, medications that promote salt retention like NSAIDs and steroids). Salt sensitivity in normotensives is associated with an increased risk for the development of hypertension, cardiovascular events, and death; therefore, dietary salt reduction should also be recommended in these persons. However, as shown in several clinical trials, long-term maintenance of low-sodium intake is difficult, even with a great deal of support, advice, and encouragement.

Other Dietary Interventions

Elderly and black hypertensives are especially sensitive to the effects of diet on BP. Multiple dietary factors have been shown to influence BP. These interventions range from whole dietary approaches to single-item nutritional modifications to the addition of dietary supplements, minerals, and vitamins. Dietary factors that increase BP and those that decrease BP are shown in Table 5-1.

The DASH Diet

The most widely accepted and recommended dietary intervention is the DASH diet. The DASH trial was a multicenter, 8-week feeding trial that

Table 5-1   Dietary Factors That May Influence Blood Pressure

Decrease Blood Pressure		Increase Blood Pressure	
• Potassium	• Protein	• Sodium chloride	• Saturated fat
• Calcium	• Fish oil	• Alcohol	• Carbohydrate
• Magnesium		• Cholesterol	

tested the effects of dietary patterns on BP. A total of 459 subjects whose average systolic BP was 120 mm Hg and average diastolic BP was 80 to 95 mm Hg were randomized into three groups: 1) control; 2) increased fruits and vegetables; and 3) combination diet that was high in fruits, vegetables, low-fat dairy products, whole grains, poultry, fish, and nuts, and that was low in fats, red meat, and sweets, after being fed a control diet for a 3-week period. The control diet was low in fruits and vegetables and dairy products, with a fat content typical of the average diet in the in the United States. Body weight and sodium intake (approximately 3 g/d) were kept constant throughout the study.

Compared with the control diet, the DASH diet had an increase in calcium content, a lower than average sodium content (3000 mg/d), 173% higher magnesium, 150% higher potassium, 240% higher fiber, and 30% higher protein. Vitamins A, B, C, and E, folate, riboflavin, phosphorus, and zinc were also higher. The participants ate whole foods, which were provided to them, and not supplements. Among nonhypertesive individuals, the DASH diet reduced systolic BP by 3.5 mm Hg and diastolic BP by 2.1 mm Hg; in hypertensives, corresponding BP reductions were 11.4 mm Hg and 5.5 mm Hg. The fruits and vegetables diet also significantly reduced systolic and diastolic BP, by 7.2 mm Hg and 2.9 mm Hg, respectively.

BP changes were evident within 2 weeks of starting the intervention feeding. After the 9-week intervention period, 70% of participants on the DASH diet had a normal BP compared with 45% on the fruits and vegetables diet and 23% on the control diet. The DASH diet reduced BP to a greater extent in African Americans than non-African Americans (20). The BP response to the DASH diet may have been a result of a balance of nutrients rather than the effect of any one nutrient.

Increased Potassium Intake

Evidence of Efficacy

Population studies examining the BP response to potassium intake have often shown an inverse relationship. A meta-analysis of 33 randomized controlled trials (n=2609) showed a 3/2 mm Hg decrease in BP for an approximate 50 mmol higher median potassium excretion, with a greater decrease in trials with 80% African Americans. The effect was enhanced in those with a high intake of sodium (18). A meta-analysis of 19 studies reveals that oral potassium supplements significantly decrease BP. The magnitude of effect is greater in patients with hypertension: on average, -8.2 mm Hg monthly systolic BP and -4.5 mm Hg monthly diastolic BP (27). Conversely, the Trials of Hypertension, Phase I (TOPH-1) study, a randomized controlled trial, showed no effect on BP from potassium supplementation over 6 months (25).

Recommendations for Clinical Practice

The preferred strategy to increase potassium intake is to consume foods rich in potassium rather than supplements. The JNC-7 recommends adoption of the DASH eating plan, which is rich in fruits, vegetables, and low-fat dairy. Potassium-rich foods include bananas, grapefruit, dried beans, peas, broccoli, spinach, pumpkin, and squash. Caution must be used by persons at risk for hyperkalemia.

Increased Calcium Intake

The effect of calcium on BP is controversial. The relationship between calcium intake and BP in both normotensives and hypertensives has been examined in meta-analyses, and the results have been inconsistent. Calcium may reduce BP in African-Americans, pregnant women, and salt-sensitive people. The proposed mechanism effect through which suboptimal calcium intake contributes to salt sensitivity and hypertension is the calciuretic effect that is exerted by a high-salt diet leading to increases in 1,25-dihydroxyvitamin D. This in turn increases vascular smooth muscle intracellular calcium, thereby increasing peripheral vascular resistance and BP. Dietary calcium reduces BP in large part via suppression of 1,25-dihydroxyvitamin D, which normalizes intracellular calcium (28).

Evidence of Efficacy

A meta-analysis of 22 clinical trials (n=1231) involving calcium supplements of 400-2160 mg/d showed a decrease in systolic BP of 1.7 mm Hg in hypertensive participants and 0.5 mm Hg in normotensive participants. Another meta-analysis of 33 trials involving calcium supplements of 1000-2000 mg/d showed a reduction in systolic BP of 1.3 mm Hg in normotensive participants. These data indicate that calcium supplementation has a small effect on systolic BP level in hypertensive persons and an uncertain effect in normotensive individuals (19).

In another meta-analysis of observational studies reported from 1983 to 1993, Preyer and colleagues found that calcium supplementation had no effect on BP (30). Similarly, in a Nurses' Health Study (normotensive subjects), there was no relationship between calcium intake and development of hypertension, nor did calcium supplementation lower BP (23).

Recommendations for Clinical Practice

Although the effect of calcium on BP is too small to justify routine use of calcium supplements specifically to prevent or treat hypertension, it remains reasonable to maintain calcium intake at recommended levels as a preventative measure against osteoporosis.

Increased Magnesium Intake

Findings associating magnesium with BP level have been inconsistent. Low dietary magnesium was found to be the dietary factor most strongly associated with high BP in the Honolulu Heart Study and the Nurses' Health Study (31). Similarly, a review of 29 observational studies concluded that the evidence suggested an inverse association between magnesium intake and BP level. However, more recent controlled clinical studies showed no significant effect of magnesium on BP (20).

Recommendations for Clinical Practice

Current guidelines recommend adoption of the DASH diet, which is rich in fruits, vegetables, and low-fat dairy products and has a reduced content of saturated and total fat and increased calcium, magnesium, potassium, and vitamins. Approximate systolic BP reduction is 8-14 mm Hg with this intervention (16). The American Heart Association Dietary Guidelines are given in Table 5-2.

Weight Reduction

Several studies have found that weight reduction has a direct beneficial effect on hypertension. Conversely, the effect of weight gain on BP has been calculated from the Framingham study, showing that for every 10% increase in relative weight, systolic BP increases by 6.5 mm Hg. Pathophysiology of obesity-related hypertension may be related to hemodynamics (increased peripheral resistance), salt sensitivity, hyperinsulinemia (anti natriuretic), and increased sympathetic nervous system activity (35). Total

---

Table 5-2   Summary of American Heart Association Dietary Guidelines

- Maintain a healthy body weight by avoiding excess total energy intake and engaging in a regular pattern of physical activity.
- Restrict total fat to less than 30% of total energy consumption, limit dietary saturated fat to less than 10% of energy, and limit cholesterol to less than 300 mg/d.
- Consume at least two fish servings per week (especially fatty fish).
- Consume a diet with a high content of vegetables and fruits (five or more servings/d) and low-fat dairy products.
- Limit sodium chloride intake to less than 6 g/d.
- For those who drink, limit alcohol (no more than two drinks/d for men and one drink/d for women).
- Consume a variety of grain products, including whole grains (six or more servings/d).

fat burden and fat distribution are important in BP elevation. Total fat burden is best assessed by calculating the body mass index (BMI) of an individual (weight in kg/height in m^2) or weight in lb/height in inches (2 × 703). The BMI correlates well with the total body fat except in very muscular individuals. A BMI of 18.5-24.9 is considered normal.

Central or upper body obesity has also been associated with increased BP in many population-based studies. Central obesity is best documented by measuring waist circumference, with greater than 102 cm in males and greater than 88 cm in women being considered abnormal by the NIH and WHO. A waste-to-hip ration has also been used with a ratio of greater than 1.0 in males and greater than .85 in women being considered abnormal. Weight-loss therapy is recommended for every overweight and obese patient with hypertension.

Evidence of Efficacy

Evidence from observational epidemiological studies has indicated that overweight is an important risk factor for hypertension. Both cross-sectional and longitudinal studies have consistently identified an association between overweight and hypertension independent of other risk factors for hypertension (21).

In the Hypertension Prevention Trial, a 4% reduction in body weight over 3 years was associated with a -2.4 mm Hg lower systolic BP and -1.8 mm Hg lower diastolic BP (22). The Trials of Hypertension Prevention (TOHP) Phase II and the Trial of Non-Pharmacological Interventions in the Elderly (TONE) examined prospectively the benefits of weight reduction alone and in combination with dietary salt reduction in individuals who were normotensive and overweight (TOHP) and hypertensive (TONE) (6,7). In the TOHP II trial, weight loss of 4 kg was associated with 2-4 mm Hg decrease in BP at 6 months. At 36 months, 2 kg weight loss was associated with approximately 1 mm Hg decrease in BP. This declining BP effect reflects poor adherence to intervention with longer follow-up (6). In the TONE study, compared with usual care, mean weight loss was approximately 10 pounds, and about one third of those in the weight-loss group were able to stop and remain off medication (7).

The long-term effects of weight loss and dietary sodium reduction on the incidence of hypertension was evaluated in the Trials of Hypertension Prevention, phase 1 (TOHP-1), a national, multi-center, randomized controlled trial. Participants were randomly assigned to one of two 18-month lifestyle modification interventions aimed at either weight loss or dietary sodium reduction or to usual care group. At baseline, subjects were 30-54 years old and had a diastolic BP of 80-89 mm Hg and a systolic BP of less than 160 mm Hg. The participants were classified as high weight (BMI 26.1-36.1 for men and 24.3-36.1 for women). Or low weight (BMI higher than 26.1 for men and lower than 24.3 for women) before randomization. Post-trial follow up analysis at 7 years was conducted in 181 participants at the Johns Hopkins clinical center. Average age was 43 years at baseline: 57% were men; 58% were white; and 46% were college graduates. At baseline, mean BP was 122/84 mm Hg, mean body weight was 81 kg, and urinary excretion of sodium was 153 mmol/24h. Baseline characteristics were similar in intervention groups and control groups. During the 18 months of active intervention, body weight decreased by 2.4 kg in the weight loss intervention group; the net difference in weight loss between the weight loss intervention and control groups was 3.5 kg. The corresponding reduction in systolic BP was 6.9 mm Hg in the intervention group and 1.2 mm Hg in the control group. The decline in diastolic BP was 8.6 mm Hg in the weight loss group and 5.5 mm Hg in the control group.

Over an average of 7 years of follow up, changes from baseline in body weight were similar in the active intervention and control groups and net changes in systolic BP and diastolic BP were -1.8 mm Hg and 1.3 Hg, respectively, in the weight loss group, compared with control group. Similarly, the incidence of hypertension was 18.9% and 40.5% in the weight loss intervention and control groups, respectively. The incidence of hypertension was 22.4% in the sodium-reduction group. This superior BP-lowering effect of weight reduction compared with sodium reduction has been demonstrated in other studies. Although their definition of normotension as lower than 160/90 mm Hg included patients with mild hypertension and their threshold for incident hypertension (lower than 160/90 mm Hg) was higher than the usual threshold of lower than 140/90 mm Hg, the results are consistent with epidemiologic evidence of the effect of weight reduction on BP.

Recommendations for Clinical Practice

The initial goal of weight loss therapy is to reduce body weight by approximately 10% to 15% from baseline. This has been shown to be achievable and maintainable with behavioral treatment and with pharmacotherapy. It is associated with significant improvements in comorbid conditions, including hypertension. Current guidelines recommend maintaining normal body weight (BMI, 18.5-24.9). Approximate systolic BP reduction is 5-20 mm Hg; 10 kg weight loss (1).

Hypertension treatment or prevention in obese patients entails a careful preliminary assessment of the patient's usual diet, habitual activity, and previous weight loss attempts (38). Psychosocial assessments should be made, and the patient's motivation should be addressed. The patient should be educated on high- and low-calorie dense foods. High-fat foods and portion sizes should be reduced, and heavy intake of sugar should be discouraged. The DASH low-sodium diet should be adopted. Alcohol should be eliminated or curtailed. The aim is for a 500 to 1000 kcal deficit for the weight loss phase and then a decreased calorie intake of approximately 30 kcal per kg for weight maintenance. Sedentary habits should be discouraged.

Physical activity may take many forms, depending on the interests and capabilities of the patient. The important parts of the exercise program are intensity, duration, and frequency, as detailed in the next section. The likelihood of weight loss maintenance is enhanced by a program consisting of dietary counseling and physical activity that is continued indefinitely. Therapy with anorectic drugs may be considered in patients with a BMI below 27, in whom a 6-month trial of diet, exercise, and behavior therapy has not proven successful.

Sibutramine and Orlistat are the only drugs that are U.S. Food and Drug Administration approved. They both have proven efficacy with weight reduction in 2-year clinical trials. However, Sibutramine, a serotonin and norepinephrine receptor reuptake inhibitor that reduces food intake by inducing early satiety, can increase BP and heart rate and is contraindicated in patients with coronary artery disease.

Orlistat is an intestinal lipase inhibitor that impairs fat absorption by the gut. The net effect is to decrease absorption of dietary fat calories. It causes steatorrhea as part of its action, with soft and more frequent loose stools. In clinical trials, over a 1-year period, 55% of Orlistat-treated patients lost more that 5% of their body weight, and 25% lost more than 10% of their body weight compared with 33% and 15%, respectively, of placebo-treated patients. Use of over-the-counter anorectic drugs should be discouraged because their safety and efficacy are generally unproven and they are not regulated. Obesity surgery may be an appropriate option in those with BMIs above 35 with very adverse health conditions. This should be done by an experienced surgical team that will commit to following the patient long-term.

Exercise

Data from epidemiologic studies indicate a strong relationship between a sedentary lifestyle and the prevalence of hypertension. Conversely, increased physical activity has been associated with lower levels of BP in observational epidemiological studies and individual clinical trials (39,40).

Exercise can be categorized into two types: aerobic and anaerobic. Aerobic exercise consists of repetitive, low-resistance movements (walking or cycling) that last over a long period of time (usually more than 10 minutes) and derive the energy source predominantly via aerobic metabolism. Anaerobic exercise consists of high-resistance, low-repetition movements such as weight lifting, and only lasts 1 to 3 minutes. Such activities derive their energy requirements predominantly from anaerobic (glycolytic) metabolism. Resistance exercise and its effect on BP has not been adequately studied.

Four characteristics of exercise are important to consider for BP lowering: frequency, duration, and length and intensity of training (44). Frequency refers to the number of sessions per week, duration refers to the length of each exercise session, and length of training refers to weeks/months required for a desirable result. Aerobic exercise has been characterized as low, moderate or high intensity by the American College of Sports Medicine. Exercise is defined as low intensity if it elicits 35%-59% of predicted maximum hear rate (PMHR), or 30%-49% of maximum oxygen uptake (Vo_2max). Moderate intensity exercise is that eliciting 60%-79% of PMHR or 50%-74% of Vo_2max (comparable to a brisk walking pace of 3 to 4 miles per hour).

Exercise eliciting a greater response is considered high intensity (comparable to jogging or running). PMHR is calculated by subtracting the patient's age from 220. For patients on medications that suppress heart rate, it is more prudent to use peak exercise heart rate achieved during a maximum exercise tolerance test. It is also prudent that all patients, regardless of age, begin exercising at low intensities. Exercise intensity should rise progressively every 2-4 weeks of regular exercise in increments of approximately 5 heartbeats.

Energy equivalents are measured in METS. One MET is the energy spent at rest to maintain body functions. Moderate intensity exercise corresponds to an equivalent of 4 METS in women and 6 METS in men. Vigorous intensity exercise corresponds to 6 METS in women and 8 METS in men.

Evidence of Efficacy

Physical activity has been associated with reduced BP in observational epidemiological studies and individual clinical trials. A meta-analysis of 54 randomized, controlled trials (n=2419) whose intervention and control groups differed only in aerobic exercise showed that aerobic exercise was associated with a significant reduction in mean systolic and diastolic BP (3.84/2.58 mm Hg)(23). A reduction in BP was associated with aerobic exercise in hypertensive and normotensive participants and in overweight and normal-weight participants. The BP reduction related to aerobic exercise did not significantly differ by subgroup according to frequency or intensity of exercise (23). The underlying mechanisms responsible for an exercise-induced reduction in BP remain unclear.

The Treatment of Mild Hypertension Study (TOMHS) showed that lifestyle modifications including weight loss and increased physical activity contribute significantly to BP control (24). These observations are supported by well-controlled exercise intervention studies, which show that regularly performed aerobic exercise of mild-to-moderate intensity lowers BP in patients with essential hypertension (43).

Convincing evidence for exercise-induced reduction of BP exits only for aerobic exercise. Besides lowering BP, regular aerobic exercise provides a number of other health benefits. Beneficial effects have been shown on the well-being index, self esteem, and overall productivity. Aerobic exercise may also improve the lipid profile, increase high-density lipoprotein cholesterol, reduce the risk of myocardial infarctions and sudden death, and eventually contributes to prolongation of life.

In a review of 12 randomized controlled trials utilizing aerobic exercise programs, lasting at least 3 months, 11 studies reported significant reduction in BP when compared with controls, but one study reported approximately 10 mm Hg systolic BP and 7.7 mm Hg in diastolic BP. The average reduction in the control group was 3.8 mm Hg and 1.3 mm Hg for systolic BP and diastolic BP, respectively, yielding a net reduction of -6.2/-6.4 mm Hg. There were no gender differences in the response of BP to exercise training.

The greater efficacy and tolerability of low to moderate exercise allows for the inclusion of older patients and those with severe hypertension in exercise studies. In a group of 70-79 year-old hypertensive patients, Cononie et al reported reductions of 8, 9, and 8 mm Hg in systolic, diastolic, and mean BP, respectively, after 6 months of aerobic exercise (45). The reductions were more modest when normotensive subjects were incuded in the analysis. This suggests that the magnitude of reduction in BP by exercise training, as with pharmacological therapy, is related to the initial level of BP.

Only a few studies have addressed the interaction of exercise training and antihypertensive medication. In one such study, 46 African-American men, ages 35-76, with severe hypertension (180/110 mm Hg) and left ventricular hypertrophy (LVH) were randomized to either usual activity or supervised aerobic program (46). Patients first entered a stabilization phase, during which they were treated with indapamide, verapamil, and enalapril as needed to reduce diastolic BP by at least 10 mm Hg or to 95 mm Hg. After 16 weeks of exercise, patients demonstrated a 7 mm Hg reduction in systolic BP and 5 mm Hg reduction in diastolic BP compared with the control group. Echocardiographic studies demonstrated that exercising patients had a 42 g reduction in LV mass ($20g/m^2$ in LV mass index). There was no change in control subjects. Exercising patients maintained lower levels of systolic BP and diastolic BP for an additional 16 weeks even though 40% of medications were discontinued. The hypotensive effect was lost 2 weeks after cessation of exercise training. This study demonstrated the benefit of regular aerobic exercise in African-American patients with treated severe hypertension.

The clinical significance of BP reduction through aerobic exercise on outcome has not been studied in long-term prospective studies. However, it is generally accepted that physical activity provides protection against cardiovascular disease. Experimental studies show that exercise training positively modifies coronary heart disease risk factors, including resting BP in hypertensive patients. The predicted reductions in mortality from stroke, coronary heart disease, and all causes are substantial, even with modest reductions in systolic BP in the entire hypertensive population. The expected reduction in stroke and coronary heart disease with .5 mm Hg reduction in diastolic BP through antihypertensive medication is about 46% and 29%, respectively. The average reduction of 10 mm Hg for systolic and 7.5 mm Hg for diastolic BP reported in the exercise studies reviewed is likely to yield similar benefits for the hypertensive patient (44).

The effectiveness of exercise in lowering BP and reducing medication requirements in patients with severe hypertension is also significant (44). LVH is considered an independent risk factor for cardiovascular disease. The risk of cardiovascular morbid events, including sudden cardiac death, increased threefold in patients with LVH. Kokkinos et al reported a 12% regression in LVH after only 16 weeks of moderate-intensity exercise (44). More favorable changes and improvement in cardiac function may be possible with longer periods of exercise training.

Recommendations for Clinical Practice

Precise exercise prescriptions for controlling BP have not been published. However, recent findings strongly suggest that low-to-moderate intensity exercise may be more effective in lowering BP than higher-intensity exercise (44). Most studies agree that most of the antihypertensive effect of aerobic exercise is achieved with 3 sessions per week. Additional periods of exercise have very little effect. The reduction of BP by low-to-moderate exercise intensities is particularly important to patients with hypertension. Low-intensity exercise as opposed to vigorous exercise carries a lower risk of injuries and cardiac complications. Patients are also more likely to participate in and continue a lower- than higher-intensity exercise program. Recommendations for exercise to control hypertension are summarized in Table 5-3.

The National High Blood Pressure Education Program recommends physical activity as an adjunctive treatment for patients with stage 2 and stage 3 hypertension and in those with stage 1 or high-normal BP who are diabetic or have demonstrable target-organ damage. It should be used as a

Table 5-3   Recommendations for Exercise Training for Prevention and Control of Hypertension*

	Pharmacotherapy	Type of Exercise	Frequency	Intensity	Duration
Mild hyper-tension	None	Brisk walk/jog; stationary bike	3-5 times per week	60%-80% of PMHR	30-60 minute session
Moderate-to-severe hyper-tension	Control BP with medication; use as adjunct therapy	Brisk walk/jog; stationary bike	3-5 times per week	50%-70% of PMHR	30-60 minute session

* All patients older than 40 years should have an exercise tolerance test to rule out coronary heart disease before engaging in a vigorous exercise program.
BP = blood pressure; PMHR = predicted maximum heart rate.
Reproduced with permission from Kokkinos PF, Narayan P, Fletcher RD, et al. Effects of aerobic training on exaggerated blood pressure response to exercise in African Americans with severe systemic hypertension treated with indapamide + verapamil + enalapril. Am J Cardiol. 1997;79:1424-6.

first-line intervention for patients with high-normal and stage 1 hypertension who are free of target organ damage and as a population-wide behavior for preventing the increase in BP that occurs with age. Numerous organizations recommend that physicians and other health care providers should counsel their patients to be physically active. All of the recommendations focus on aerobic exercise as the primary activity. Some of the recommendations include weight training as part of an overall fitness regimen, but none recommend weight training as a sole mode of exercise.

Resistance exercise and its effect on BP has not been adequately studied. Current guidelines recommend engaging in regular aerobic physical activity such as brisk walking at least 30 minutes per day, most days of the week. Approximate systolic BP reduction is 4-9 mm Hg for this intervention (16).

Moderation of Alcohol Consumption

Alcohol consumption has paradoxic effects on the cardiovascular system, with a J-shaped risk profile for alcohol intake reflecting the protective effect of small amounts of alcohol against coronary atheroma. Many epidemiologic studies have shown a direct relationship between alcohol intake and hypertension, especially above an average intake of two drinks per day (48).

Several mechanisms have been proposed for the relationship between alcohol and elevated BP, and the real mechanism remains debatable. An immediate effect of alcohol ingestion is vasodilation in some vascular beds. Sustained intake accompanied by high blood-alcohol levels results in short-term elevation of BP. BP levels usually correlate best with alcohol intake within the previous 24 hours, and BP levels fall within hours to days after cessation or reduction in intake. This suggests that the effects on BP may be mediated by reversible physiologic changes rather than structural alterations. Suggested mediators include stimulation of the sympathetic nervous system, endothelin, rennin-angiotensin-aldosterone system, insulin resistance, corticotrophin, or cortisol, inhibition of vascular-relaxing substances such as nitric oxide, calcium depletion, magnesium depletion, increased intracellular calcium or other electrolytes in vascular smooth muscle, and increased acetaldehyde. However, there is some evidence that hypertension in frequent heavy drinkers is mediated by a chronic state of alcohol withdrawal.

Evidence of Efficacy

The Pitt County study, a longitudinal investigation since 1988 of hypertension predictors among 970 African Americans aged 25 to 50 years, showed a strong hypertension gradient for alcohol consumption and BP for both men and women (49). The mean increase in systolic BP among persons who initiated alcohol consumption during the study was 6.2 mm Hg greater than among abstainers; persons who reported drinking at the study beginning and continued had a rise in BP of 3.8 mm Hg greater than abstainers. Increase in BP for persons who discontinued drinking were comparable with those of abstainers. The initiation and continuation of alcohol consumption was significantly associated with social and economic factors.

A meta-analysis of 15 randomized controlled trials (n=2234) in which alcohol reduction was the only intervention difference between active and control treatment groups (26). Overall, alcohol reduction was associated with a significant reduction in mean systolic and diastolic BPs of 3.31/2.04 mm Hg. A dose-response relationship was observed between mean percentage of alcohol reduction and mean BP reduction. Effects of intervention were enhanced in those with higher baseline BP (50). Although the majority of these studies included relatively few subjects, were of short duration, and were not designed as effectiveness trials, the results are consistent with epidemiologic evidence on the relationship of alcohol with BP.

Patterns of alcohol consumption may be associated with other cardiovascular consequences. In persons with pre-existing coronary artery disease, binge drinking can lead to silent myocardial ischemia and angina. It has been hypothesized that binge drinking may induce cerebrovascular spasm or cause ventricular and supraventricular arrhythmias, especially atrial fibrillation. In other randomized controlled trials, the reduction of BP seen from reducing alcohol intake is comparable with or quantitatively greater than the differences found for most of the other lifestyle interventions.

Recommendations for Clinical Practice

All hypertensive patients should be asked about recent drinking, including quantity and frequency of drinking. Those who drink should be given appropriate screening for alcohol dependence. Effective interventions such as the cognitive-behavioral technique used in PATHS trial have been developed to reduce alcohol consumption in nondependent heavy drinkers (51). Referral to alcohol treatment specialists is necessary in many cases, if there is evidence of alcohol dependence or more serious health consequences.

Current guidelines recommend limitation of alcohol consumption to no more than two drinks per day (1 oz or 30 mL ethanol; e.g., 24-oz beer, 10-oz wine, or 3-oz 80-proof whiskey) in most men and no more than 1 drink per day in women and lighter-weight persons. Approximate systolic BP reduction with this intervention is 2-4 mm Hg (16).

Relaxation Techniques and Biofeedback

The role of stress in the development and maintenance of hypertension is unsettled. Some evidence of an association has accumulated in findings that job stress in particular may lead to long-term BP elevations (53). In a longitudinal study of job strain and ambulatory BP among 215 men, an effect on systolic ambulatory BP of cumulative past exposure to job stress plus current exposure was shown (54). Those with 50% of their employment lifetime (average: 25 years) exposed to job strain as well as current job strain had 10.7 mm Hg higher work systolic ambulatory BP and 15.4 mm Hg systolic ambulatory BP than those with no current or past exposure. Short-term studies have found applied stress to be associated with short-term increases in BP.

Studies suggest that chronic stress-induced sympathetic nervous system stimulation causes hypertension via neuroendocrine responses (27). Early studies by Patel reported large falls in BP in patients who took part in relaxation, with or without biofeedback (28).

Johnston pooled the results of all randomized trials involving stress management and concluded that stress management doubles the fall in BP compared with controls (29). In contrast, the large trials of the Hypertension Prevention Study found no effect on BP from stress management (30).

Recommendations for Clinical Practice

Currently there is insufficient evidence to advocate stress management as a useful strategy for the prevention of hypertension. In a subset of patients with hypertension and chronic anxiety disorder, BP may not be fully controlled until the anxiety is controlled. In this setting, anxiety management with supportive psychotherapy and coping skills may be beneficial.

Conclusions

Lifestyle modifications decrease BP, enhance antihypertensive drug efficacy, and, as a result, decrease cardiovascular risk. Adoption of healthy lifestyles by all individuals is critical for the prevention of high BP and is an indispensable part of the management of those with hypertension. Nonpharmacologic interventions should include sodium restriction, weight loss, a diet high in fruit and vegetables (the DASH diet), and regular aerobic exercise. Combinations of two or more lifestyle modifications can achieve additive results (16). Overall the benefit varies from patient to patient, but, on average, reductions in BP as much as 15/10 mm Hg can be expected. If nonpharmacologic interventions are not adequate within a period of 3-6 months, pharmacologic therapy is appropriate. The major limitation of nonpharmacologic interventions is poor adherence. Persons with a genetic predisposition may respond to these interventions differently. Thus, in practice, lifestyle modifications and nonpharmacologic interventions will work for a small number of patients, and these changes are very effective for the prevention of hypertension. Most patients with moderate-to-severe hypertension will require a combination of nonpharmacologic interventions and pharmacologic therapies.

◼ ◼ ◼

Key Points

- Increased physical activity, weight loss, reduced dietary sodium, moderate alcohol intake, and adoption of a diet rich in fruits, vegetables, nuts, and low-fat dairy, and low in sweets and cholesterol, are lifestyle modifications that have proven benefits in BP reduction.

- The DASH low sodium diet and weight reduction approach has proven efficacy, particularly in older hypertensive persons and African Americans; patients should be cautioned about the sodium content in processed foods.

- In hypertensive persons, lifestyle changes can serve as initial treatment before the start of drug therapy and may facilitate drug step-down or drug withdrawal in highly motivated persons.

- In non-hypertensive persons, lifestyle changes can prevent hypertension and thus lower cardiovascular risk, especially in salt-sensitive individuals.

- Lifestyle changes may be difficult to achieve and maintain; therefore, emphasis should be on developing strategies to implement and sustain these interventions.

◼ ◼ ◼

REFERENCES

1. **Chobanian AV, Bakris GL, Black HR, et al.** The Seventh Report of the Joint National Committee on Prevention, Detection, Evaluation, and Treatment of High Blood Pressure. JAMA. 2003;289:2560-71.

2. **Chobanian AV, Hill M.** National Heart, Lung, and Blood Institute Workshop on Sodium and Blood Pressure: a critical review of current scientific evidence. Hypertension. 2000;35:858.

3. **Lewington S, Clarke R, Qizilbash N, et al.** Age-specific relevance of usual blood pressure to vascular mortality: a meta-analysis of individual data for one million adults in 61 prospective studies. Lancet. 2002;360:1903-13.

4. **Neal B, MacMahon S, Chapman N.** Effects of ACE inhibitors, calcium antagonists, and other blood-pressure-lowering drugs: results of prospectively designed overviews of randomized trials. Lancet. 2000;356:1955-64.

5. The Fifth Sir George Pickering Memorial Lecture. Epitaph to essential hypertension: a preventable disorder of known aetiology? J Hypertens. 1988;6:85-94. Review.

6. **Tobian L.** Lessons from animal models that relate to human hypertension. Hypertension. 1991;17(Suppl I):I-52-I-58.

7. **He J, Tell GS, Tang YC, et al.** Relation of electrolytes to blood pressure in men. Hypertension. 1991;17:378-85.

8. **Denton D, Weisinger R, Mundy NI, et al.** The effect of increased salt intake on blood pressure of chimpanzees. Nat Med. 1995;1:1009-16.

9. The Trials of Hypertension Prevention Collaborative Research Group. Effects of weight loss and sodium reduction intervention on blood pressure and hypertension incidence in overweight people with high-normal blood pressure: the Trials of Hypertension Prevention, Phase II. Arch Intern Med. 1997;157:657-67

10. **Whelton PK, Appel LJ, Espeland MA, et al** for the TONE Collaborative Research Group. Efficacy of sodium reduction and weight loss in the treatment of hypertension in older persons: main results of the randomized, controlled trial of nonpharmacologic interventions in the elderly. JAMA. 1998;279:839-46.

11. **Sacks FM, Svetkey LP, Vollmer WM, et al** for the DASH-Sodium Collaborative Research Group. Effects on blood pressure of reduced dietary sodium and the Dietary Approaches to Stop Hypertension (DASH) diet. N Engl J Med. 2001;344: 3-10.

12. **Vollmer WM, Sacks FM, Ard J, et al.** Effects of diet and sodium intake on blood pressure: subgroup analysis of the DASH-sodium trial. Ann Intern Med. 2001;135: 1019-28.

13. **Stamler J, Rose G, Stamler R, et al.** INTERSALT study findings: public health and medical care implications. Hypertension. 1989;14:570-7.

14. **Alderman MH, Madhavan S, Ooi WL, et al.** Low urinary sodium is associated with greater risk of myocardial infarction among treated hypertensive men. Hypertension. 1995;25:1144-52.

15. **Tunstall-Pedoe H, Woodward M, Tavendale R, et al.** Comparison of the prediction by 27 different factors of coronary heart disease and death in men and women of the Scottish Heart Health Study: cohort study. BMJ. 1997;315:722-9.

16. **Alderman MH, Cohen H, Madhavan S.** Dietary sodium intake and mortality: the National Health and Nutrition Examination Survey. Lancet. 1998;351:781-5.

17. **Cohen JD, Grandis G, Cutler JA, et al.** Dietary sodium intake and mortality: MRFIT Follow-up Study results. Circulation. 1999;100(Suppl I):I-524.

18. **Graudal NA, Galloe AM, Garred P.** Effects of sodium restriction on blood pressure, renin, aldosterone, catecholamines, cholesterols, and triglyceride: a meta-analysis. JAMA. 1998;279:1383-9.

19. **MacGregor GA, Sever PS.** Salt-overwhelming evidence but still no action: can a consensus be reached with the food industry? BMJ. 1996;312:1287-9.

20. **Conlin PR, Chow D, Miller III ER, et al** for the DASH Research group. The effect of dietary patterns on blood pressure control in hypertensive patients: results from the Dietary Approaches to Stop Hypertension (DASH) trial. Am J Hypertens. 2000; 13:949-55.

21. **Whelton PK, He J, Cutler JA, et al.** Effects of oral potassium on blood pressure: meta-analysis of randomized clinical trials. JAMA. 1997;277:1624-32.

22. **Stamler J.** Blood pressure and high blood pressure. Aspects of risk. Hypertension. 1991;18(Suppl): I95-I107.

23. **Sacks FM, Willett WC, Smith A, et al.** Effect on blood pressure of potassium, calcium, and magnesium in women with low habitual intake. Hypertension. 1998; 31:131-8.

24. **Ascherio A, Hennekens C, Willett WC, et al.** Prospective study of nutritional factors, blood pressure, and hypertension among US women. Hypertension. 1996;27: 1065-72.

25. Trials of Hypertension Prevention Collaborative Research Group. The effects of nonpharmacologic interventions on blood pressure of persons with high normal levels: results of the Trials of Hypertension Prevention Phase 1. JAMA. 267;1992: 1213-20.

26. **Brancati FL, Appel LJ, Seidler AJ, et al.** Effect of potassium supplementation on blood pressure in African Americans on a low-potassium diet: a randomized, double-blind, placebo-controlled trial. Arch Intern Med. 1996;156:61-7

27. **Cappuccio FP, Macgregor GA.** Does potassium supplementation lower blood pressure? A meta-analysis of published trials. J Hypertens. 1991;9:465-73.

28. **Zemel MB.** Calcium modulation of hypertension and obesity: mechanisms and implications. J Am Coll Nutr. 2001;20(5 Suppl):428S-35S. Discussion: 440S-2S.

29. **Allender PS, Cutler JA, Follmann D, et al.** Dietary calcium and blood pressure: a meta-analysis of randomized clinical trials. Ann Intern Med. 1996;124:825-9.

30. **Pryer J, Cappuccio FP, Elliott P**. Dietary calcium and blood pressure: review of the observational studies. J Hum Hypertens. 1995;9:597-604.

31. **Beilin LJ, Puddey IB, Burke V.** Lifestyle and hypertension. Am J Hypertens. 1999; 12:934-45.

32. **Mizushima S, Cappuccio FP, Nichols R, Elliott P.** Dietary magnesium intake and blood pressure: a qualitative overview of the observational studies. J Hum Hypertens. 1998;12:447-53.

33. **Yamamoto ME, Applegate WB, Klag MJ, et al.** Lack of blood pressure effect with calcium and magnesium supplementation in adults with high-normal blood pressure: results from Phase I of the Trials of Hypertension Prevention (TOPH). Ann Epidemiol. 1995;5:96-107.

34. **Kannel WB, Brand N, Skinner JJ Jr, et al.** The relation of adiposity to blood pressure and development of hypertension: the Framingham Study Ann Intern Med. 1967;67:48-59.

35. **Landsberg L.** Obesity. In: Izzo JL, Black HR, eds. Hypertension Primer. 3rd ed. Philadelphia: Lippincott Williams Wilkins; 2003:129-31.

36. **Cassano PA, Segal MR, Vokonas PS, Weiss ST.** Body fat distribution, blood pressure, and hypertension: a prospective cohort study of men in the normative aging study. Ann Epidemiol. 1990;1:33-48.

37. **He J, Whelton PK, Appel LJ, et al.** Long-term effects of weight loss and dietary sodium reduction on incidence of hypertension. Hypertension. 2000;35:544.

38. National Heart, Lung, and Blood Institute. Clinical guidelines on the identification, evaluation, and treatment of overweight and obesity in adults: the evidence report. Obes Res. 1998;6:51S-209S.

39. National High Blood Pressure Education Program Working Group. Prevention of hypertension. Arch Intern Med. 1993;153:186-208.

40. World Hypertension League, Physical exercise in the management of hypertension: a consensus statement by the world hypertension league. J Hypertens. 1991;9:283-7.

41. **Whelton SP, Chin A, Xin X, He J.** Effect of aerobic exercise on blood pressure: a meta-analysis of randomized, controlled trials. Ann Int Med. 2002;136:493-503.

42. **Grimm RH, Grandits GA, Cutler JA, et al.** Relationships of quality-of-life measures to long-term lifestyle and drug treatment in the treatment of mild hypertension study. Arch Intern Med. 1997;157:638-48.

43. **Akinpelu AO.** Responses of the African hypertensive to exercise training: Preliminary observations. J Hum Hypertens. 1990;4:74-6.

44. **Papademetriou V, Kokkinos P.** Exercise training and blood pressure control in patients with hypertension. J Clin Hypertension. 1999;1:95-105.

45. **Cononie CC, Graves JE, Pollock ML, et al.** Effect of exercise training on blood pressure in 70-79 year-old men and women. Med Sci Sports Exerc. 1991;23:505-11.

46. **Kokkinos PF, Narayan P, Fletcher RD, et al.** Effects of aerobic training on exaggerated blood pressure response to exercise in African-Americans with severe systemic hypertension treated with indapamide + verapamil + enalapril. Am J Cardiol. 1997;79:1424-6.

47. **Motoyama M, Sunami Y, Kinoshita F, et al.** Blood pressure lowering effect of low intensity aerobic training in elderly hypertensive patients. Med Sci Sports Exerc. 1998;30:818-23.

48. **Puddey IB, Beilin LJ, Vandongen R, et al.** Hypertension. 1985;7:707-13.

49. **Curtis AB, James SA, Strogatz DS, et al.** Alcohol consumption and changes in blood pressure among African Americans: the Pitt County Study. Am J Epidemiol. 1997;146:727-33.

50. **Xin X, He J, Frontini MG, et al.** Effects of alcohol reduction on blood pressure: a meta-analysis of randomized controlled trials. Hypertension. 2001;38:1112.

51. **Cushman WC, Cutler JA, Hanna E, et al** for the PATHS Group. The prevention and treatment of hypertension study (PATHS): effects of an alcohol treatment program on blood pressure. Arch Intern Med. 1998;152:1197-207.

52. **Rakic V, Puddey IB, Burke V, et al.** Influence of pattern of alcohol intake on blood pressure in regular drinkers: a controlled trial. J Hypertens. 1998;16:165-74.

53. **Kaplan NM.** Clinical Hypertension, 7th ed. New York: Williams & Wilkins: 1997.

54. **Schnall PL, Schwartz JE, Landsbergis PA, et al.** A longitudinal study of job strain and ambulatory blood pressure: results from a three-year follow-up. Psychosom Med. 1998;60:697-706.

6

■   ■   ■

Pharmacology of
Antihypertensive Drugs

L. Michael Prisant, MD

ardiovascular and renal disease account for the major morbidity and mortality of hypertension. However, with the knowledge of the principles of antihypertensive drug pharmacology, most patients can be easily treated. The search for the "perfect antihypertensive" drug has resulted in the proliferation of a large number of blood pressure (BP)–lowering medications. However, tailoring treatment using appropriate drugs with outcome data within a drug class makes the task of drug selection easier.

BP control is a lifetime endeavor. Factors of efficacy and patient adherence are key components in attaining current treatment recommendations. Combinations of antihypertensive drugs are often required because BP control is not achieved by monotherapy in most patients. Adherence to drug therapy is a function of dosing frequency, side effects, cost, and many other factors. Using low-dose, fixed-dose combination therapy reduces dose-dependent side effects and maximizes BP control.

General Principles

Treatment Goals

The BP target for hypertensive patients with diabetes mellitus and chronic renal insufficiency is below 130/80 mm Hg, and with proteinuria in excess of one gram over 24 hours is less than 125/75 mm Hg (1). For all other patients, the treatment goal is less than 140/90 mm Hg. To achieve BP control, most patients will require more than one drug (Figure 6-1).

Lifestyle modification is recommended for all patients with hypertension regardless of whether they are treated with drugs. The closer the patient is

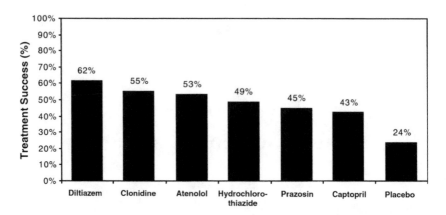

Figure 6-1 Blood pressure control with monotherapy. Treatment success is defined as a diastolic blood pressure less than 90 mm Hg at the end of the titration period and after 1 year of treatment. The placebo-corrected control rate for each antihypertensive drug is less than 50%. (Modified from data from Reference 9.)

to the goal of treatment, the more likely it is that nonpharmacologic therapy will be effective without drug treatment. It should be remembered that the lifetime risk for drug treatment is quite high.

Factors in Drug Selection

Drug characteristics to consider when selecting an agent include mode of action, route of elimination, and potential drug interactions. An additional factor for drug selection is knowledge of outcomes trials because one should not assume that each drug within a drug class has a "class effect" in protecting or reducing hypertensive target-organ damage. Patient factors such as age, gender, race, and concomitant diseases (Table 6-1) are important in drug selection. For example, β-blockers and angiotensin-converting enzyme (ACE) inhibitors are less effective in black patients than in white patients. Initially, older patients respond better to diuretics and calcium channel blockers (CCB) than ACE inhibitors. As another example, the glomerular filtration rate of a patient may require reduction of the drug dose or avoidance of the drug.

Additionally, it is wise to select an initial drug that can treat more than one disease process: for example, a β-blocker to treat both hypertension and angina due to coronary ischemia. A further example is using an ACE inhibitor to treat a patient with both heart failure and diabetes.

Patients with secondary hypertension require a different approach. An aldosterone-secreting tumor would be treated with spironolactone or eplerenone. Hyperthyroidism requires a nonselective β-blocker such as propranolol. A pheochromocytoma should be treated with an α_1-blocker initially while avoiding β-blockers and diuretics. An ACE inhibitor may control BP in a patient with unilateral renal artery stenosis with two kidneys.

Table 6-1   Potential Drug Choices for Common Co-morbidities

Compelling Indication	ACE Inhibitor	Aldosterone Antagonist	ARB	β-blocker	CCB	Diuretic
Chronic kidney disease	✓		✓			
Diabetes mellitus		✓		✓	✓	✓
Heart failure	✓	✓	✓	✓		✓
High CAD risk	✓			✓	✓	✓
Prior myocardial infarction	✓	✓		✓		
Recurrent stroke	✓					✓

Modified from the Seventh Report of the Joint National Committee (1).
Abbreviations: ACE = angiotensin converting enzyme; ARB = angiotensin receptor blocker; CCB = calcium channel blocker; CAD = coronary artery disease.

Monotherapy controls BP in fewer than 50% of patients with hypertension. Patients who are close to the target BP are easily treated with a single drug. The higher the BP, the more likely that more than one drug will be required. Black and diabetic hypertensives commonly require two or more drugs for BP control, whereas patients with chronic renal insufficiency need three or more drugs.

Dosing Strategies and Drug Efficacy

A low dose of drug may be started initially with stage I hypertension or in fragile elderly patients. The BP is reassessed in 4 to 6 weeks. At that visit, the patient is monitored for drug-specific side effects. If the BP medication is well tolerated and the BP is uncontrolled, then the drug must be further titrated or a second drug added.

As the dose of a drug is doubled, additional BP-lowering decrements diminish (Figure 6-2). Drug monotherapy, even when titrated, will achieve a placebo-corrected control rate of less than 50% (Figure 6-1). Furthermore, as a drug dose is increased, there is a higher rate of dose-dependent side effects (Figure 6-2). For example, as the dose of a dihydropyridine CCB is increased, the likelihood of peripheral edema increases. However, not all side effects are dose-dependent; some drugs (e.g., ACE inhibitors) have dose-independent side effects such as cough or angioneurotic edema. Thus, the dominant benefit of drug therapy balanced against adverse events is within about two titrations. Drug titrations should occur after 4 to 6 weeks.

Generally, drugs are selected that are dosed once daily or twice daily. Adherence to therapy diminishes when drugs are dosed more frequently. Ideally, one should synchronize the dosing of antihypertensive medications with other medications.

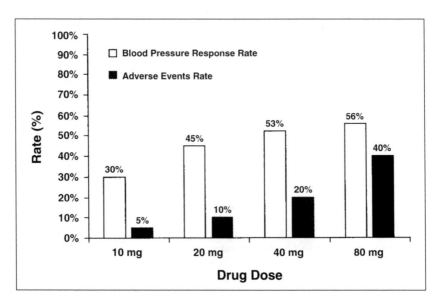

Figure 6-2 Relationship of drug dose: response rate and side effects. As the drug dose increases, the increment in response rate to doubling the dose diminishes; however, side effects increase progressively.

The effectiveness of a drug at a given dose can be diminished by other medications. For example, excess sodium intake or nonsteroidal anti-inflammatory agents (NSAIDs) (e.g., ibuprofen, celecoxib) will reduce the effectiveness of most antihypertensive drugs.

Not all antihypertensive drugs are additive to one another, but diuretics tend to augment all antihypertensive agents. Drugs that combine different pharmacologic mechanisms increase the chance of attaining treatment goals. Fixed-dose combinations offer some financial advantages and convenience for patients.

Drug Classes

A wide variety of drugs are available for the treatment of hypertension:

- diuretics
- β-blockers
- CCBs
- ACE inhibitors
- angiotensin-receptor blockers (ARBs)

- α_2-stimulants
- α_1-blockers
- peripheral sympatholytics
- direct vasodilators

Peripheral sympatholytics are not used frequently. There is a place for the use of low-dose reserpine, as a part of a low-cost combination with a diuretic for patients who have no access to other medications. α_2-stimulants (e.g., clonidine), peripheral sympatholytics, and direct vasodilators (hydralazine and minoxidil) are not considered first-line therapy for the treatment of hypertension. α_1-blockers (prazosin, terazosin, and doxazosin) have fallen out of favor as initial therapy for hypertension, but have been safely used for many years.

When there were fewer drugs, a stepped-care approach was used to achieve target BPs. Now individual-tailored therapy is a more common approach. However, an algorithm approach using a rational combination of antihypertensive medications is likely to manage a diastolic BP 90% and systolic BP 70% of the time.

Diuretics

Mode of Action and Pharmacology

There are three classes of diuretics used for hypertension: thiazide or thiazide-like, loop, and potassium-sparing diuretics. All diuretics are secreted into the urine by the proximal tubule cells (2).

Thiazide (e.g., hydrochlorothiazide) and *thiazide-like diuretics* (e.g., chlorthalidone, indapamide, and metolazone) work initially by increasing urinary sodium excretion by inhibiting the sodium-chloride pump in the early segment of the distal convoluted tubule. This causes is an initial reduction in plasma volume, which increases plasma renin activity and aldosterone. Eventually, vascular resistance decreases by unknown mechanisms because plasma volume approaches pretreatment levels.

Loop diuretics include furosemide, bumetanide, torsemide, and ethacrynic acid. Loop diuretics act at the thick ascending loop of Henle to prevent chloride and sodium reabsorption from the urine. They have a rapid onset of action compared with thiazide diuretics. Torsemide is the longest-acting loop diuretic.

There are four *potassium-sparing diuretics:* amiloride, triamterene, spironolactone, and eplerenone. They are often used in combination with hydrochlorothiazide. Potassium-sparing diuretics decrease excretion of magnesium and potassium. Spironolactone is a potent nonselective aldosterone blocker that also interacts with androgen and progesterone receptors. Eplerenone is a selective aldosterone blocker. Both amiloride and triamterene block epithelial sodium transport channel. Unlike spironolactone and eplerenone, they do not significantly reduce BP.

Clinical Use

The treatment of hypertension was revolutionized with the discovery of diuretics in the 1950s. Thiazide or thiazide-like diuretics are proven therapy for reducing strokes, heart failure, or total cardiovascular mortality. Outcome trials have established their benefit for both isolated systolic hypertension and diastolic hypertension. Hydrochlorothiazide is prescribed most often, although chlorthalidone has been used in many clinical trials. The recommended dose of diuretics has decreased over the last 10 years in order to decrease the metabolic side effects. A fixed-dose combination of a thiazide diuretic and potassium-sparing diuretic is used to diminish the potassium and magnesium wasting.

Diuretics are especially effective for obese, African-American, elderly, and diabetic patients. They are often required for patients who have systolic heart failure and excess sodium intake. Thiazide diuretics are known to increase calcium and decrease osteoporosis. Diuretics are avoided in patients who have severe recurrent gout, hyponatremia, or volume depletion.

Loop diuretics are ineffective treatment for hypertensive patients with normal renal function. Generally loop diuretics should be used in patients whose serum creatinine exceeds 2.5 mg/dL. In heart failure, furosemide has been shown to have an acute venodilator affect, when given intravenously. Ethacrynic acid is the only non-sulfonamide diuretic. However, it is associated with permanent ototoxicity at high doses.

Spironolactone reduces mortality and morbidity in advanced heart failure. Eplerenone decreases total and cardiovascular mortality in patients who sustained a myocardial infarction with left ventricular dysfunction. Eplerenone is expected to be useful in the treatment of African Americans and patients with resistant hypertension and diabetes mellitus.

Drug Combinations

All other drug classes are additive to thiazide diuretics. Metolazone can be added to a loop diuretic if the patient becomes refractory to its diuretic effect. Diuretics are a necessary component of a triple combination with direct vasodilators. Diuretic effectiveness is reduced with the use of NSAIDs, including COX-2 inhibitors (celecoxib, rofecoxib).

Side Effects

The side effects of thiazide diuretics include volume depletion, hyponatremia, hypokalemic alkalosis, hypomagnesemia, hypercalcemia, hyperuricemia, gout, sexual dysfunction, and occasionally sulfonamide-related skin eruptions (3). Volume depletion and hyponatremia are more likely to occur with high doses of a diuretic, vomiting, diarrhea, or excessive heat exposure. Hyponatremia occurs in some elderly patients even when a low dose of diuretics is used; therefore, careful monitoring is necessary. Failure to replete potassium may decrease their effectiveness in cardiovascular-event reduction. However, this continues to be an issue that is controversial. Lipid abnormalities occur transiently, but this does not preclude their use (4). There is an increased risk of the development of diabetes mellitus with diuretics (12% versus 8%) compared with the ACE inhibitors (5). Side effects of loop diuretics are similar to thiazide diuretics, except hypocalcemia may occur.

The major potential problem with potassium-sparing diuretics is hyperkalemia. Hyperkalemia can occur in patients with renal insufficiency, diabetes mellitus, and type IV renal tubular acidosis or with concomitant use of potassium supplements, over-the-counter salt substitutes, ACE inhibitors, ARBs, and NSAIDs. Triamterene is associated with megaloblastic anemia, due to folic acid antagonism, and nephrolithiasis. Amiloride is associated with nausea, diarrhea, and headache. Spironolactone in high doses causes erectile dysfunction, gynecomastia, mastodynia, and menorrhagia. Eplerenone is not associated with these side effects because it has a lower affinity for the androgen and progesterone receptors.

β-Blockers

Mode of Action and Pharmacology

There are three β-receptors: $β_1$ in the myocardium, kidney, and adipose tissue; $β_2$ in smooth and skeletal muscle, liver, pancreas, salivary glands, and lungs; and $β_3$ in brown adipose tissue and striated muscle for lipolysis and thermogenesis. Stimulation of $β_1$-receptors increases heart rate, myocardial contractility, renin release, lipolysis, and antidiuretic hormone release. $β_2$-receptor stimulation relaxes smooth muscle, including bronchioles, and increases amylase, insulin secretion, glycogenolysis, and gluconeogenesis.

β-blockers are a heterogenous group of drugs from pharmacologic point of view, but they all share the ability to block the receptors for norepinephrine. Their antihypertensive mechanism of action is not entirely certain. β-blockers are known to increase peripheral vascular resistance acutely, inhibit renin release (Figure 6-3) and decrease the vasoconstrictor angiotensin II, reduce heart rate, and decrease cardiac output (6). Because β-blockers reduce BP, it is postulated that they have a central nervous system mechanism.

It is convenient to sort β-blockers according to various characteristics (Figure 6-4): elimination route, intrinsic sympathomimetic activity, $α_1$-blocking characteristics, membrane stabilizing activity, and $β_1$-selectivity (7). The liver metabolizes lipophilic β-blockers. Hydrophilic β-blockers, which include atenolol, nadolol, sotalol, and carteolol, are renally eliminated; thus, the dose must be reduced with renal insufficiency. β-blockers with intrinsic sympathomimetic activity (acebutolol, carteolol, labetalol, pindolol, and penbutolol) have vasodilating characteristics. These drugs are less likely to cause bradycardia, claudication, and alterations in lipids. Two β-blockers, labetalol and carvedilol, possess $α_1$-blocking characteristics, which cause vasodilation. They are effective in the elderly and black patients and do not affect the glomerular filtration rate (7). They also may be advantageous for

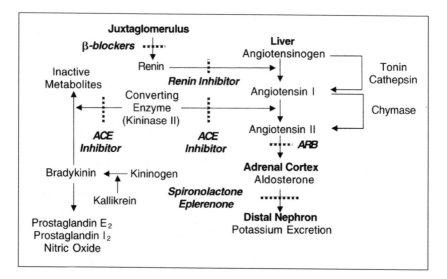

Figure 6-3   Blockade of the renin angiotensin aldosterone system. β-blockers block the release renin. ACE inhibitors block the action of the converting enzyme on angiotensin I and bradykinin. ARBs block the action of angiotensin II at the receptor. The aldosterone blockers are spironolactone and eplerenone.

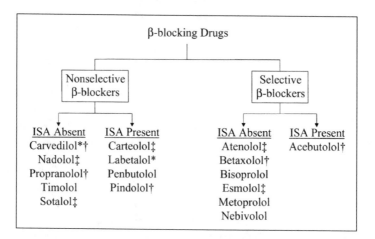

Figure 6-4   Pharmacologic properties of β-blockers. The pharmacologic properties of β-blockers are shown (see text for further description). ISA = intrinsic sympathomimetic activity; * α_1-blocker; † Membrane-stabilizing activity; ‡ Hydrophilic.

hypertensive patients with insulin resistance. β-blockers possessing membrane-stabilizing activity may contribute to antiarrhythmic activity. Also, carvedilol has a potent antioxidant effect. Intravenous β-blockers include atenolol, esmolol, metoprolol tartrate, and labetalol.

β_1-selectivity is a characteristic associated with less bronchospasm and claudication in low doses. The selective β-blockers include acebutolol, atenolol, betaxolol, bisoprolol, esmolol, metoprolol tartrate, metoprolol succinate, and nebivolol. However, no β-blocker is cardioselective in large doses. β_2-blockade is necessary for essential tremor and migraine headaches. β_1-blockers are better for bronchospastic pulmonary disease, peripheral vascular disease, and diabetes mellitus (7).

Clinical Use

Despite the de-emphasis of β-blockers for the initial therapy of hypertension, the combination of β-blockers and diuretics for the treatment of elderly hypertensive patients reduced total mortality. Specific β-blockers have been proven useful for the treatment of hypertension, myocardial infarction, heart failure, hypertrophic cardiomyopathy, and arrhythmias. Given these pharmacologic differences, using individual β-blockers can be confusing. However, if drugs are selected on the basis of outcome studies, then the choices become easier. For instance, timolol, metoprolol tartrate, propranolol, acebutolol, and carvedilol are protective after a myocardial infarction. Bisoprolol, carvedilol, and metoprolol succinate (but not metoprolol tartrate) decrease mortality in heart failure. Both atenolol and bisoprolol improve cardiovascular outcomes in the perioperative period. Metoprolol succinate reduces carotid atherosclerosis.

All currently marketed β-blockers have an indication for hypertension except for sotalol, which is used as an antiarrhythmic drug. β-blockers tend to be less effective in African Americans compared with whites (8). However, when β-blockers are used in combination with diuretics, there is no difference in BP response. There is a belief that these drugs are not effective in elderly patients because there is reduced activity of the renin-angiotensin system; however, the Veterans Affairs Cooperative Study Group on Antihypertensive Agents study in men does not support that conclusion (9). Younger patients, especially those that are more anxious or have hyperkinetic heart syndrome, also benefit from β-blockers. Essential tremor and migraine headaches are helped by nonselective β-blockers. β-blockers decrease the ventricular response rate of atrial fibrillation and other supraventricular tachycardias. They are an important adjunct to therapy with patients who are receiving concomitant direct vasodilators. β-blockers are considered standard necessary therapy for all patients who have sustained a myocardial infarction and have heart failure (10,11). Their use in heart failure should not be initiated until the patient's symptoms are stable and fluid excess has been resolved.

Drug Combinations

β-blockers are additive to diuretics and α_1-blockers, but they are not additive to ACE inhibitors for augmenting an antihypertensive effect (12). β-blockers should not be added to α_2-stimulants (e.g., clonidine). Abrupt withdrawal of either drug causes a marked elevation in BP due to unopposed α-receptor–induced vasoconstriction. Combining verapamil or diltiazem with a β-blocker increases the risk of myocardial depression, extreme bradycardia, and advanced heart block. However, this combination could be cautiously used in patients with hyperkinetic heart syndrome or hypertrophic cardiomyopathy. Dihydropyridine CCBs are added to β-blockers for the treatment of angina that is refractory to monotherapy.

Side Effects

Although not supported by randomized trials, there have been a number of side effects associated with β-blockers (13). These include depression and erectile dysfunction (3). Some weight gain is common with these drugs. There is a predictable increase in the triglyceride level and a reduction in HDL cholesterol (4). Special care should be used in combining nonselective β-blockers for patients with insulin-dependent diabetes mellitus because symptoms of hypoglycemia can be masked and there can be a hypertensive response to hypoglycemia. Abrupt discontinuation of β-blockers can result in withdrawal symptoms that can be dangerous in the presence of coronary artery disease. A slow tapering over a 14-day period or longer is advisable.

Angiotensin-Converting Enzyme Inhibitors

Mode of Action and Pharmacology

Angiotensin II is a potent direct vasoconstrictor (14). Angiotensin II also augments cardiac output by amplifying sympathetic activity, increases thirst and antidiuretic hormone secretion, stimulates the adrenal cortex to release aldosterone, and acts on the kidney to increase sodium reabsorption. Angiotensin II directly decreases renin release. Angiotensin II has potent cellular growth properties, resulting in vascular and cardiac hypertrophy. Many tissues and organs can synthesize angiotensin II, independent of the classic circulating system.

ACE inhibitors work by inhibiting ACE or kininase II (Figure 6-3). Inhibition of ACE prevents conversion of angiotensin I to angiotensin II and the breakdown of bradykinin (14). Angiotensin I can be converted to angiotensin 1-9 by ACE 2 in the heart and kidney. Angiotensin 1-9 is converted by ACE to angiotensin 1-7, which is a vasodilator.

It should be noted that there are other pathways by which angiotensin II is generated (Figure 6-3). Thus, angiotensin II levels will return toward baseline levels even with the use of ACE inhibitors. However, there are additional benefits of ACE inhibitors that may influence the observed antihypertensive effects, including an increase in vasodilating bradykinin, prostacyclin (prostaglandin I2) and nitric oxide, a reduction in aldosterone secretion, inhibition of the sympathetic nervous system, suppression of endothelin, and venodilation. Reflex tachycardia does not occur.

Several characteristics differentiate ACE inhibitors. Three different zinc-binding ligands allow the ACE inhibitors to attach to the converting enzyme (15). All ACE inhibitors use a carboxylic zinc-binding ligand, except for captopril, which uses a sulfhydryl group, and fosinopril, which uses a phosphinyl group. All ACE inhibitors, except captopril and lisinopril, are prodrugs, which improve the rate of absorption and remain inactive until converted by the liver (14). For example, enalapril is converted to enalaprilat. Prodrugs are not an issue for selection unless advanced impaired hepatic function is present. Most ACE inhibitors are renally excreted; thus, the dose is reduced in the setting of renal failure. An exception is fosinopril and trandolapril, which have a dual hepatic and renal excretion. Tissue ACE inhibition is a characteristic of quinapril, benazepril, ramipril, perindopril, and trandolapril. Although ACE inhibitors may differ according to their binding affinity for tissue ACE, the clinical significance remains to be determined. Lipophilicity is another characteristic that has not been proven therapeutically important. The most lipophilic ACE inhibitors include fosinopril, captopril, ramipril, trandolapril, and quinapril. Trandolapril, ramipril, perindopril, and lisinopril are the longest-acting ACE inhibitors. Captopril should be dosed 2 to 3 times per day. The others may be dosed once or twice daily. Intravenous enalaprilat is available. Food reduces the absorption of captopril and moexipril.

Clinical Use

ACE inhibitors approved for the treatment of hypertension are listed in Table 6-2. Although only enalapril is proven to reduce systolic heart failure mortality, captopril, enalapril, fosinopril, lisinopril, quinapril, ramipril, and trandolapril are approved for heart failure. Enalapril is indicated for asymptomatic left ventricular dysfunction. Captopril, lisinopril, ramipril, and trandolapril are designated for left ventricular dysfunction after myocardial infarction. Ramipril is specified for prevention of myocardial infarction, stroke, and cardiovascular death.

Despite low levels of plasma renin, elderly patients respond as well as younger patients to ACE inhibitors (9). ACE inhibitors are less effective in African Americans compared with whites. Higher doses of an ACE inhibitor improve the hypotensive effect. However, when ACE inhibitors are combined with the diuretics they are equally effective for blacks and whites. In African Americans, if hypertensive renal insufficiency is present, ramipril is superior to amlodipine or metoprolol, as a part of a multiple-drug regimen, in slowing glomerular filtration rate decline. ACE inhibitors delay the development of renal failure in type II hypertensive diabetics with microalbuminuria (16). ACE inhibitors decrease the rate of renal failure progression in patients with renal insufficiency due to type I diabetes and nondiabetic nephropathy.

Table 6-2   Angiotensin Converting Enzyme Inhibitors and Indications for Specific Agents

Drug	Trade Name	Dose	Other Indications Based on Outcome Trials
Benazepril	Lotensin	10-80 mg in 1-2 doses	Chronic renal insufficiency
Captopril	Capoten	12.5-150 mg in 2-3 doses	Post-myocardial infarction Type I diabetic kidney disease
Enalapril	Vasotec	2.5-40 mg in 1-2 doses	Heart failure
Fosinopril	Monopril	10-80 in 1-2 doses	
Lisinopril	Prinivil/Zestril	5-40 mg in 1 dose	Post-myocardial infarction
Moexipril	Univasc	7.5-30 mg in 1-2 doses	
Perindopril	Aceon	4-8 mg in 1-2 doses	Post-myocardial infarction Recurrent stroke (with indapamide)
Quinapril	Accupril	5-80 mg in 1-2 doses	
Ramipril	Altace	1.25-20 mg in 1-2 doses	Post-myocardial infarction Nondiabetic kidney disease Hypertensive nephrosclerosis in blacks Vascular diseases protection
Trandolapril	Mavik	1-8 mg in 1-2 doses	Post-myocardial infarction

ACE inhibitors are also used for scleroderma renal crisis. In addition they reduce the rate of development of diabetes. ACE inhibitors are indicated as a necessary part of therapy for patients with coronary artery disease and heart failure (10,11).

Drug Combinations

ACE inhibitors may be combined with most drugs, especially diuretics and CCBs. However, there is only a marginal antihypertensive effect in combination with a β-blocker (12). Combining maximum doses of an ACE inhibitor and angiotensin-receptor blocker is not proven to provide additional BP reduction. NSAIDs attenuate the BP-lowering effect of ACE inhibitors.

Side Effects and Contraindications

If ACE inhibitors are initiated in the presence of high renin levels, volume depletion, or diuretics, hypotension may occur (14). Captopril is associated with dermatologic eruptions and dysgeusia. Rarely, ACE inhibitors cause cholestatic jaundice and pancreatitis. Neutropenia and agranulocytosis occur with high doses of captopril in patients with renal insufficiency or autoimmune disorders.

The most common side effects of ACE inhibitors include intractable cough, hyperkalemia, deteriorating creatinine, and angioneurotic edema. Reversible renal insufficiency with ACE inhibitors arises in patients who have bilateral renal artery stenosis, renal artery stenosis in a solitary kidney, or extrinsic compression of the renal arteries with polycystic kidney disease (17). Creatinine increases also with underlying renal disease, heart failure, volume depletion, sepsis, and use of NSAIDs, cyclosporine, and tacrolimus. ACE inhibitors reduce intrarenal angiotensin II, causing a vasorelaxant effect on the efferent arteriole, reducing glomerular pressure. An increase of creatinine of 20% to 30% is acceptable because this indicates that intraglomerular pressure is successfully reduced (17). If the increase in creatinine is greater than 30% and confirmed, then the ACE inhibitor should be stopped and the cause for the increase determined. Hyperkalemia is most likely to occur in patients receiving NSAIDs, potassium-sparing diuretics, potassium supplements, and in patients with renal insufficiency, diabetes mellitus, and type IV renal tubular acidosis (14). Cough is a non-dose-dependent side effect of ACE inhibitors affecting up to 10% of patients. This usually is not improved by switching to another ACE inhibitor.

Angioneurotic edema (Figure 6-5) is an unpredictable side effect that is more likely to occur among African Americans than whites. The risk is three times higher among African Americans (5). Angioedema usually affects the face but can also involve the hands, feet, genitalia, and bowel. Laryngeal edema is life threatening and requires a hospital admission. ACE inhibitors are contraindicated during pregnancy. Miscarriage can occur if ACE inhibitors are used during the second and third trimester. An additional contraindication is in patients with bilateral renal artery stenosis or unilateral stenosis with a solitary kidney.

Angiotensin Receptor Blockers

Mode of Action and Pharmacology

Angiotensin II receptors are located in the brain, heart, kidney, adrenal gland, and blood vessels (18). The role of angiotensin II is to defend the body acutely against hemorrhage or dehydration. However, chronic effects are ventricular and vascular hypertrophy. ARBs block the type I angiotensin II (AT1) receptor, which mediates vasoconstriction. Once the AT1 receptor is blocked, plasma renin, angiotensin I, and angiotensin II increase. There are other angiotensin II receptor subtypes, but the AT2 receptor is present during fetal development. The AT2 receptor may mediate apoptosis and tissue remodeling (19). Stimulation of AT2 receptors from blockade of the AT1 receptor increases nitric oxide production and afferent arteriolar dilatation.

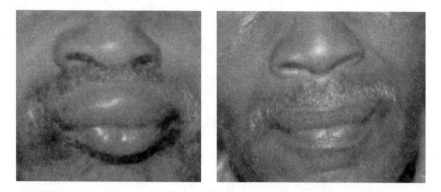

Figure 6-5   Angioneurotic edema. Angioneurotic edema of the upper and lower lips is present during treatment with an ACE inhibitor in the left panel. The right panel shows the resolution of the angioedema.

ARBs available for the treatment of hypertension are listed in Table 6-3. Losartan and its active E3174 metabolite reduce BP. Candesartan cilexetil and olmesartan medoxomil are prodrugs that form an active metabolite. Losartan has a uricosuric effect. Food decreases the absorption of valsartan. Telmisartan has the longest terminal half-life. Olmesartan, valsartan, candesartan, irbesartan, and telmisartan are insurmountable antagonists of angiotensin II.

Clinical Use

ARBs work equally well in young and older patients. However, ARBs are less effective in African Americans, but these differences are overcome with a low dose of a diuretic. ARBs are indicated in hypertensive type II diabetic patients with macroalbuminuria (>300 mg/d), nephropathy, or renal insufficiency, and in patients with heart failure who are intolerant to ACE inhibitors (11,16). Like ACE inhibitors, ARBs delay the progression to macroalbuminuria in hypertensive type II diabetic patients with microalbuminuria (16).

Outcome trials with ARBs continue to be reported. Losartan decreased the rate of development of renal failure in patients with diabetic nephropathy. In hypertensive patients with left ventricular hypertrophy, losartan, compared to the β-blocker atenolol, reduced the rate of stroke and, among diabetic patients, decreased total mortality and cardiovascular mortality. The rate of development of diabetes was lower with losartan compared with atenolol. Irbesartan reduced the rate of doubling the serum creatinine compared with placebo or amlodipine in type II diabetics with renal insufficiency. Valsartan decreased hospitalization rates in heart failure patients treated with an ACE inhibitor compared with placebo, but did not reduce mortality. Candesartan decreased all-cause mortality and cardiovascular

Table 6-3   Angiotensin Receptor Blockers and Indications for Specific Agents

Drug	Trade Name	Dose	Other Indications Based on Outcome Trials
Candesartan	Atacand	8-32 mg in 1 dose	Heart failure mortality
Eprosartan	Teveten	400-800 mg in 1-2 doses	
Irbesartan	Avapro	150-300 mg in 1 dose	Type II diabetic nephropathy
Losartan	Cozaar	25-100 mg in 1-2 doses	Type II diabetic nephropathy Hypertension with left ventricular hypertrophy
Olmesartan	Benicar	20-40 mg in 1 dose	
Valsartan	Diovan	80-320 mg in 1 dose	Heart failure hospitalizations, post-infarction left ventricular dysfunction
Telmisartan	Micardis	40-80 mg in 1 dose	

deaths in patients with heart failure and reduced hospitalization rates. Candesartan decreased stroke rates in elderly hypertensives.

Drug Combinations

ARBs are additive to diuretics; however, there are scanty data on combination with other antihypertensive drugs. There is an interest in combining ACE inhibitors and ARBs for renal protection.

Side Effects and Contraindications

ARBs are one of the best-tolerated classes of antihypertensive drugs. Side effects are similar to placebo. Cough is not seen, and angioedema is rare. However, increases in serum creatinine and hyperkalemia can occur (19). Like ACE inhibitors, ARBs are contraindicated in pregnancy.

Calcium Channel Blockers

Mode of Action and Pharmacology

CCBs (or calcium antagonists) represent one of the most popular drug classes used for hypertension. The CCBs (Table 6-4) are divided into three classes: dihydropyridine (nifedipine and others), benzothiazepine (diltiazem), and phenylalkylamine (verapamil).

All CCBs block the transmembrane flux of calcium from the outside to the inside of the cell, causing vasodilatation. The CCBs bind to the $\alpha_1 c$

Table 6-4   Indications for Calcium Antagonists

Generic/Brand Name	Stable	Vasospastic Angina	Hypertension Angina	Supraventricular Tachycardia
Benzothiazepine				
Diltiazem/Cardizem	✓	✓		✓
Diltiazem/Cardizem-SR			✓	
Diltiazem/Cardizem-CD	✓	✓	✓	
Diltiazem/Cardizem LA*			✓	
Diltiazem/Dilacor-XR	✓		✓	
Diltiazem/Tiazac			✓	
Dihydropyridine				
Amlodipine/Norvasc	✓	✓	✓	
Felodipine/Plendil			✓	
Isradipine/DynaCirc	✓		✓	
Isradipine/DynaCirc-CR			✓	
Nicardipine/Cardene	✓		✓	
Nicardipine/Cardene-SR			✓	
Nifedipine/Adalat/Procardia	✓	✓		
Nifedipine/Adalat CC			✓	
Nifedipine/Procardia XL	✓	✓	✓	
Nisoldipine/Sular			✓	
Phenylalkylamine				
Verapamil/Calan/Isoptin	✓	✓	✓	✓
Verapamil/Calan-SR			✓	
Verapamil/Covera-HS*	(		✓	
Verapamil/Isoptin-SR			✓	
Verapamil/Verelan			✓	
Verapamil/Verelan-PM†			✓	

* Chronotherapeutic delivery system.

subunit of the L-type channel (20). L-type channels are located on cardiac muscle, arteries, and veins. In addition, they are situated on leukocytes, platelets, brain, retina, salivary glands, gastric mucosa, pancreas, adrenal glands, pituitary gland, and other smooth muscle (bronchial, gastrointestinal, genitourinary, and uterine). Other effects of CCBs that potentially lower BP include acute and repetitive natriuresis, inhibition of aldosterone, and interference with α_2-mediated with angiotensin II–mediated vasoconstriction.

Most people prefer to simply divide the CCBs into dihydropyridines, which are vasodilating, and nondihydropyridines, which are myocardial active, to emphasize their relative vascular to cardiac selectivity action. Diltiazem reduces sinoatrial conduction time slightly. Both verapamil and diltiazem decrease conduction through the AV node and reduce myocardial contractility. Dihydropyridines have a dose-dependent negative inotropic effect, but this is offset by systemic vasodilation.

The dihydropyridine CCBs include amlodipine, felodipine, isradipine, lercanidipine, nicardipine, nifedipine, nimodipine, and nisoldipine. All dihydropyridines other than nifedipine, lacidipine, and lercanidipine are referred to second-generation dihydropyridines. The third-generation dihydropyridines are lercanidipine and lacidipine, which are hydrophobic, membrane soluble, and have a long duration of action (21). Tissue selectivity refers to a ratio, calculated as a 50% inhibition of vascular constriction versus inhibition of the contractility of isolated myocardium (22). The higher the ratios are, the more selective the CCB is for vascular tissue and the lower the potential is for producing a negative inotropic effect. The most selective is nisoldipine. Intermediate selectivity is observed with felodipine, isradipine, and nicardipine. The lowest tissue selectivity among the dihydropyridines is observed with nifedipine and amlodipine.

Most CCBs have a short duration of action. Only amlodipine and lercanidipine have a long half-life. The remaining CCBs use drug-delivery systems to prolong their duration of action (23). There are three CCBs that are chronotherapeutic formulations. The delivery systems are dosed at 10:00 p.m. and achieve their highest concentrations throughout the early morning hours, when most cardiovascular events occur.

Clinical Use

Although this drug class has been controversial for the initial treatment of hypertension, recent data do not support an increase in coronary heart disease events or total mortality (5,7,24). CCBs are generally effective for all age groups and equally effective in whites and blacks (9). In the elderly, the elimination is prolonged compared with younger patients (20). Interestingly, although gender has not been viewed as a factor in the response of antihypertensive agents, there are data to suggest that verapamil is not cleared as well and plasma concentrations are higher in women. Although high sodium intake and NSAIDs attenuate the antihypertensive effect of other drugs, the CCBs are somewhat resistant to this attenuation.

There are specific areas in which CCBs are proven useful. The dihydropyridine nitrendipine reduced stroke and blunt cognitive decline in elderly patients with isolated systolic hypertension. Verapamil reduces reinfarction rate after myocardial infarction. Also, a modest antiatherosclerotic effect has been demonstrated. Diltiazem decreases reinfarction rate after nontransmural myocardial infarction.

CCBs should be avoided in the setting of an acute myocardial infarction or unstable angina, although it is valuable for cocaine-induced vasospasm.

CCBs are contraindicated in patients with systolic heart failure (11). Although not tested prospectively, there may be a beneficial role in patients who have heart failure, characterized by a normal ejection fraction and a diastolic filling abnormality. Dihydropyridines are not protective against renal failure in African Americans and diabetics with advanced renal insufficiency when compared with ARBs or ACE inhibitors. However, diabetic patients who are pretreated with an ARB or an ACE inhibitor appear to be safe. Dihydropyridines lower cardiovascular events in diabetics with isolated systolic hypertension. Nondihydropyridines in smaller studies reduce proteinuria like ACE inhibitors, but outcome trials do not exist. CCBs are effective in cyclosporin-induced hypertension.

An intravenous form of nicardipine exists for hypertensive emergencies. Amlodipine, diltiazem, nicardipine, nifedipine, and verapamil are approved for stable angina. Diltiazem and verapamil are available in an intravenous formulation. Both diltiazem and verapamil have an indication for atrial fibrillation, atrial flutter, and paroxysmal supraventricular tachycardia. Nimodipine is not indicated by hypertension, but is used for subarachnoid hemorrhage. Because CCBs improve smooth muscle relaxation in nonvascular and vascular tissues, they are used for esophageal spasm, primary pulmonary hypertension, Raynaud's phenomenon, and migraine headaches.

Drug Combinations

Most drugs are additive to CCBs. There is some controversy concerning the effectiveness of adding a diuretic in patients receiving a CCB. Fixed-dose combinations are available with a CCB and an ACE inhibitor. Even dihydropyridine and nondihydropyridine CCBs seem to be additive. The combination of a CCB with an α_1-blocker may be synergistic; thus, one has to be very careful and slowly titrate the α_1-blocker to avoid extreme hypotension. A dihydropyridine should be chosen for the CCB combination with a β-blocker to avoid bradycardia, advanced heart block, and heart failure.

Care must be taken when combining nondihydropyridines with other drugs that slow the heart rate such as digitalis preparations, amiodarone, flecainide, disopyramide, and α_2-stimulants. There are a number of drug-drug interactions with CCBs, especially verapamil and diltiazem; thus, it is critical that all drugs be recognized before initiating drug therapy (20).

Side Effects

Verapamil causes constipation as a dose-dependent side effect. Rarely, heart block or skin eruptions can occur. Sinus bradycardia, peripheral edema, headache, dizziness, asthenia, fatigue, and rash occur with diltiazem. Short-acting dihydropyridines trigger vasodilator side effects, including flushing and tachycardia; however, this occurs less commonly with long-acting dihydropyridines.

Dihydropyridines produce dose-dependent peripheral edema. This is not the result of salt and water retention, but it is caused by precapillary arterial vasodilatation and relative venular constriction. This is diminished by concomitant use of an ACE inhibitor. All CCBs can cause gingival overgrowth (Figure 6-6), like cyclosporin or phenytoin (25). Esophageal reflux is more likely to develop with CCBs.

The drug-delivery systems used with CCBs require special knowledge (23). For instance, felodipine, nifedipine, and nisoldipine use a hydrophilic gel surrounding active drug to prolong the duration of action. Dividing the tablet causes a sudden release of the drug, causing flushing, headache, and tachycardia. The gastrointestinal delivery system, used with nifedipine, isradipine, and verapamil, should not be used in patients who have diverticula or stenosis anywhere in the gastrointestinal tract because these tablets are quite hard and can cause obstruction or erosion.

α1-Blockers

Mode of Action and Pharmacology

α_1-receptors are located postsynaptically on vascular smooth muscle cells (26). Norepinephrine interacts with the α_1-receptors to cause vasoconstriction. α_1-blockers reverse the vasoconstrictive effects of norepinephrine and epinephrine (27). As a consequence of selective α_1-blockade, there is a

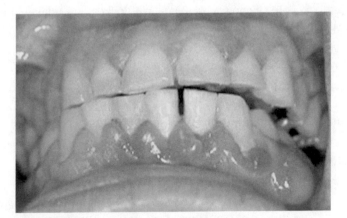

Figure 6-6   Gingival growth associated with calcium antagonists. The gingival changes occur with calcium antagonists, cyclosporine, and phenytoin. It results in pain, gingival bleeding, and periodontal disorders. (Reproduced with permission from Prisant LM, Herman W. Calcium channel blocker induced gingival overgrowth. J Clin Hypertens (Greenwich). 2002;5:310-1.)

decrease in BP with no important decrease in cardiac output or increase in heart rate or norepinephrine levels. There is both venous and arterial dilatation. Modest sodium and water retention can occur (27).

Oral phenoxybenzamine and intravenous phentolamine are nonselective α-blockers because they block both presynaptic and postsynaptic α-receptors. Phenoxybenzamine is a noncompetitive blocker, and phentolamine is a competitive blocker. Both of these drugs are used in the management of pheochromocytoma or catecholamine excess states.

The selective α_1-blockers are currently used for treating hypertension include prazosin, terazosin, and doxazosin. Doxazosin has the longest duration of action. The β-blockers that possess concomitant α-blocking qualities include labetalol and carvedilol.

Clinical Use

Selective α_1-blockers can be effectively used to treat hypertension, but their role as initial antihypertensive therapy has fallen into disfavor. The Antihypertensive and Lipid-lowering Treatment to Prevent Heart Attack Trial reported a higher rate of heart failure and stroke with doxazosin compared with the diuretic chlorthalidone (28). Systolic BP control was not equivalent between the two groups. However, there was no difference in fatal and nonfatal myocardial infarction rate.

These drugs reduce constriction of the urinary sphincter and decrease symptoms of prostatism by increasing urinary flow. α_1-blockers have the best metabolic profile of any class of antihypertensive drug by decreasing LDL cholesterol and triglycerides, increasing HDL cholesterol, and improving glucose uptake into muscle (29). Thus, they are less likely than diuretics or β-blockers to precipitate diabetes. α_1-blockers are unlikely to cause erectile dysfunction (3).

Drug Combinations

These drugs are very effective for achieving BP control as a part of a multidrug regimen. α_1-blockers are additive with all drug classes, except α_2-stimulants. α_1-blockers appear to be synergistic with CCBs.

Side Effects and Contraindications

Hypotension or syncope may happen in the presence of volume depletion (27). The dose must be gradually titrated to effect and the BP monitored in the upright posture to avoid hypotension. If the drug is stopped and not titrated again, profound dizziness or syncope can occur. Although selective α_1-blockers are beneficial for prostatism, they should be avoided in patients with stress urinary incontinence. Asthenia and nasal congestion occur. Rarely, priapism is reported.

Central α_2-Stimulants

Mode of Action and Pharmacology

α-methyldopa, clonidine, guanabenz, and guanfacine are the central α_2-stimulants (central sympatholytics or α-agonists). These drugs reduce sympathetic outflow from the nucleus tractus solitarii and rostral ventrolateral medulla; therefore, these drugs would not be effective in patients with the spinal cord transection. Inhibition of sympathetic nerve activity and norepinephrine release causes blood vessels to dilate (30). Plasma norepinephrine and renin activity decrease (31). High doses of central α_2-stimulants can actually increase BP by stimulating peripheral α_2-receptors (31).

Unlike the other α-agonists, α-methyldopa is a prodrug that is converted to α-methylnorepinephrine, which stimulates the central α_2-adrenoreceptors. In addition, clonidine also stimulates the I1-imidazoline receptor. Selective I1-imidazoline receptor agonists, moxonidine and rilmenidine, decrease BP with fewer side effects than α_2-stimulants. I1-imidazoline receptors are located in rostral ventrolateral medulla, hypothalamus, and renal proximal tubule (30).

Clinical Use

The central α_2-stimulants are not used for initial therapy for the treatment of hypertension due to salt and water retention, referred to as pseudotolerance, because the sympathetic nervous system is not activated. This class is effective for most patient groups, including African Americans and the elderly. These drugs should not be used in patients who are poorly adherent to treatment.

Because α-agonists preserve renal blood flow and do not diminish the glomerular filtration rate, they are frequently used in patients undergoing hemodialysis. The dose of clonidine and methyldopa need to be reduced with renal insufficiency. Guanfacine is the longest-acting oral α_2-stimulant. A 7-day transdermal clonidine preparation is available that can be used in the perioperative period for patients who are not able to take oral medications. However, it takes three days to achieve adequate blood levels. Methyldopa remains an important adjunct for treatment during pregnancy-induced hypertension.

Drug Combinations

α_2-stimulants are additive to diuretics, but they are not additive to α_1-blockers or β-blockers. The combination of a β-blockers and an α_2-stimulant is risky because cessation of either drug results in unopposed vasoconstriction. Tricyclic antidepressants antagonize the BP reduction with this drug class.

Side Effects

Sedation, erectile dysfunction, and dry mouth occur commonly with α-agonists. The dry mouth can promote dental caries and periodontal disease. Due to a sudden surge in catecholamines, patients who suddenly stop taking these drugs have a rapid return of their BP to the pretreatment level or even higher levels within 24 to 36 hours (32). Tachycardia, tremulousness, and anxiety may also occur. This discontinuation syndrome is magnified with concomitant β-blocker therapy.

These drugs lower heart rate to a variable degree and should be cautiously used in combination with other drugs that reduce heart rate or in sick sinus syndrome. The major limitation of the clonidine patch is skin irritation or an allergic skin reaction. Also hyperpigmentation and depigmentation of the skin occur. Methyldopa is associated with hepatotoxicity and Coombs' positive hemolytic anemia. Galactorrhea occurs occasionally with methyldopa.

Peripheral Sympatholytics

Mode of Action and Pharmacology

The peripheral sympatholytics include rauwolfia alkaloids (reserpine, deserpidine, rauwolfia serpentina), guanadrel, and guanethidine. Peripheral sympatholytics block the transport of norepinephrine into storage granules at the postganglionic sympathetic nerve ending (33). When the adrenergic nerve is stimulated, less norepinephrine is available for vasoconstriction. Central nervous system catecholamines are depleted with reserpine, a mechanism of action that is not shared by guanethidine and guanadrel.

Clinical Use

These drugs are rarely used today. When used in doses less than 0.1 mg per day in combination with a diuretic, reserpine is effective, inexpensive, and well tolerated. Guanethidine and guanadrel are no longer used.

Side Effects

Reserpine in higher doses is associated with nasal stuffiness, depression, and increased gastric acidity. Low doses of reserpine are unlikely to cause depression (34). Guanethidine and guanadrel side effects are attributable to sympathetic blockade and include orthostatic symptoms, frequent bowel movements or diarrhea, bradycardia, reduced cardiac output, and retrograde ejaculation.

Direct Vasodilators

Mode of Action and Pharmacology

There are two direct vasodilators, hydralazine and minoxidil (35,36). The mechanism by which these drugs reduce BP is not known, but they dilate resistance and capacitance vessels. They lose their effectiveness when given as monotherapy because they reflexively increase renin, norepinephrine, and cardiac output, and cause salt and water retention (Figure 6-7). Minoxidil is the most potent oral vasodilator.

Clinical Use

The direct vasodilators are the drugs of last resort for refractory treatment of hypertension. They are never used as monotherapy. These drugs always require a diuretic and a drug such as verapamil, diltiazem, reserpine, α_2-stimulant, or β-blocker to block the reflex increase in heart rate. Thus they are usually a part of a triple-drug regimen (36).

Hydralazine and minoxidil can be a part of a low-cost antihypertensive regimen. Hydralazine is used safely during pregnancy. Hydralazine and nitrates may be used for heart failure in patients who are intolerant of ACE inhibitors or have advanced renal failure precluding the use of an ACE inhibitor or ARB (11). Minoxidil is used in patients with refractory hypertension or in patients with chronic renal insufficiency.

Side Effects

Hydralazine is inactivated in the liver by acetylation. The rate of acetylation is genetically determined by the activity of hepatic N-acetyltransferase. Among

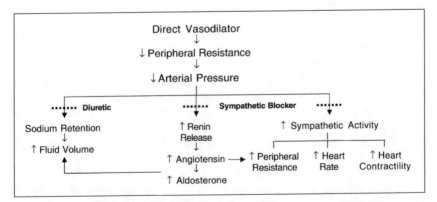

Figure 6-7   Compensatory mechanisms of tolerance of direct vasodilators. Direct vasodilators reduce peripheral vascular resistance, causing tachycardia, renin and aldosterone release, and salt and water retention, which increases blood pressure to pretreatment levels. A diuretic and a sympathetic blocker prevent the consequences of the compensatory mechanisms.

fast acetylators, higher doses of hydralazine may be used. Toxicity of this drug occurs more commonly with slow acetylators (35). The major risk of hydralazine is a lupus-like reaction, characterized by arthralgias, weight loss, splenomegaly, and pleural and pericardial effusions. It happens most commonly in doses greater than 200 mg per day. Drug fever, anemia, leukopenia, thrombocytopenia, and neuropathy due to pyridoxine deficiency also occur. Intravenous hydralazine results in flushing, tachycardia, and headache. It should not be given to patients with ischemic heart disease.

Minoxidil causes fluid retention and hypertrichosis, making this cosmetically unacceptable for women (36). Pericardial effusions have also been reported.

Optimal Use Strategies

Demographics

The selection of the initial antihypertensive drug therapy is based on age, race, target organ damage, and coexisting illnesses. Figure 6-8 displays the diastolic BP control rate according drug, age, and race (9). For example, older white patients are similarly controlled with each drug class tested, whereas younger and older black patients are best controlled with diltiazem and hydrochlorothiazide. In general, women and men do not respond differently to antihypertensive therapy; however, there may be differences in response to specific drugs. For instance, because verapamil plasma concentrations are higher in women, there is a greater reduction in BP. Women who are likely to become pregnant should not be given ACE inhibitors or ARBs because of the risk of birth defects.

Coexisting Illnesses

The selection of drugs based on co-morbidities is a higher priority than selection based on age and race. Based on the patient's comorbidities, the most appropriate agents can be selected to prevent compromise of specific target organs. For example, ACE inhibitors are indicated in patients with type 1 and type 2 diabetes to delay progression of chronic kidney disease; in nondiabetic patients with chronic kidney disease to preserve renal function; in patients with heart failure; in patients with a myocardial infarction; and for recurrent stroke prevention. Aldosterone antagonists may be considered in patients with heart failure and myocardial infarction with left ventricular dysfunction. A full discussion of drug selection based on improving specific cardiovascular outcomes is given in Chapter 7 and is summarized in Table 7-4 of that chapter.

An understanding of the outcome trial and of the population tested will provide optimal information for decision making for patients. For example, chlorthalidone and nitrendipine (not available in the United States) are

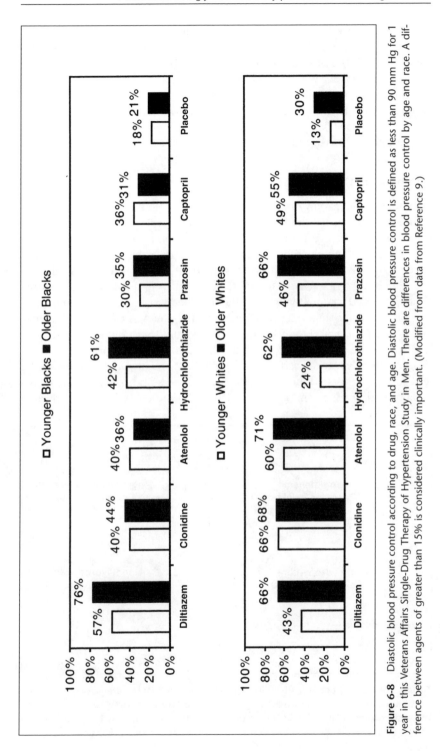

Figure 6-8   Diastolic blood pressure control according to drug, race, and age. Diastolic blood pressure control is defined as less than 90 mm Hg for 1 year in this Veterans Affairs Single-Drug Therapy of Hypertension Study in Men. There are differences in blood pressure control by age and race. A difference between agents of greater than 15% is considered clinically important. (Modified from data from Reference 9.)

proven to reduce cardiovascular morbidity in older patients with isolated systolic hypertension; however, additional drugs were required to reach the target BP (37,38). For instance, in the Syst-Eur Trial, the goal was to achieve a target BP in elderly patients with isolated systolic hypertension. Active treatment for initial titration was nitrendipine 10 to 40 mg with the potential addition of enalapril 5 to 20 mg and hydrochlorothiazide 12.5 to 25 mg to attain the prespecified target BP. Thus, this was not a trial of monotherapy that resulted in stroke reduction.

Combination Drugs for Treatment

Monotherapy alters only one of several pathophysiological components of BP. Figure 6-1 emphasizes the fact that most patients will require more than one medication to achieve BP control. Systolic BP control is more difficult than diastolic control. An algorithm treatment approach has been used successfully to meet the BP treatment goals in clinical trials (5,39,40). If the initial drug after titration did not achieve the BP target, then second- and third-line drugs could be added for titration to meet the treatment goals. Diuretics are usually required to be a component of the treatment regimen. A two-drug combination is usually required for a BP level 160/100 mm Hg or higher (Figure 6-9).

Drug-induced compensatory mechanisms favor combining certain drugs. Diuretics activate renin due to volume contraction; β-blockers, ARBs, and ACE inhibitors counter this effect. β-blockers and α_2-stimulants cause sodium and water retention that is offset with diuretic use. The natriuretic

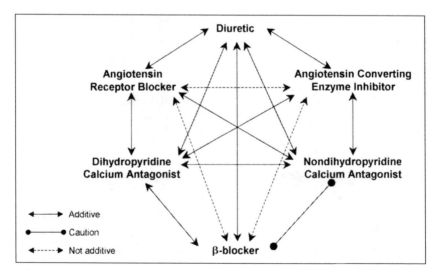

Figure 6-9   Blood pressure–lowering effects of first-line drugs used in combination. Drugs are added in sequence to achieve a target blood pressure. However, not all antihypertensive drugs are additive with each other. Despite this, there may be reasons to add drugs in combination that are not additive to achieve target organ protection.

effect of CCBs enhances the antihypertensive effect of ACE inhibitors, which reduces the dihydropyridine-induced peripheral edema. However, not all drugs are additive with each other: ACE inhibitors (and probably ARBs) and β-blockers, β-blockers and α_2-stimulants, and α_2-stimulants and α_1-blockers.

Fixed-dose combinations are available with: 1) diuretics and CCBs, ACE inhibitors, ARBs, β-blockers, or central α_2-stimulants, and 2) ACE inhibitors and CCBs. The use of fixed-dose combination drugs requires knowledge of their individual components. Useful combinations allow physicians to titrate the individual components to achieve BP control.

Future Therapy

Oral renin inhibitors, endothelin antagonists, selective I1-imidazoline receptor agonists and vasopeptidase inhibitors are classes of antihypertensive drugs that may be added to our treatment armamentarium in the future. The recognition that combination therapy will be required for most patients will expand therapeutic options with more fixed-dose multidrug combination products for clinicians and patients.

■ ■ ■

Key Points

- Select initial antihypertensive drug therapy based on age, race, target organ damage, and coexisting illnesses.
- Assess potential drug-related side effects before initiating therapy and during follow-up visits.
- Titrate the initial drug choice once or twice at 4- to 6-week intervals.
- Add rational, additional antihypertensive medications to achieve BP treatment goals.
- Target a BP of 130/80 mm Hg for patients with diabetes mellitus and chronic kidney disease and 140/90 mm Hg for all other individuals.
- Assess all over-the-counter and prescribed (including ophthalmic drugs) medications for possible pharmacokinetic and pharmacodynamic interactions with antihypertensive drugs.

■ ■ ■

REFERENCES

1. **Chobanian AV, Bakris GL, Black HR, et al.** The Seventh Report of the Joint National Committee on Prevention, Detection, Evaluation, and Treatment of High BP: the JNC 7 report. JAMA. 2003;289:2560-72.

2. **Brater DC.** Diuretic therapy. N Engl J Med. 1998;339:387-95.

3. **Grimm RH, Jr., Grandits GA, Prineas RJ, et al.** Long-term effects on sexual function of five antihypertensive drugs and nutritional hygienic treatment in hypertensive men and women. Treatment of Mild Hypertension Study (TOMHS). Hypertension. 1997;29(1 Pt 1):8-14.

4. **Weir MR, Moser M.** Diuretics and beta-blockers: is there a risk for dyslipidemia? Am Heart J. 2000;139(1 Pt 1):174-83.

5. Major outcomes in high-risk hypertensive patients randomized to angiotensin-converting enzyme inhibitor or calcium channel blocker vs diuretic: The Antihypertensive and Lipid-Lowering Treatment to Prevent Heart Attack Trial (ALLHAT). JAMA. 2002;288:2981-97.

6. **Man in 't Veld AJ, Schalekamp MA.** Effects of 10 different beta-adrenoceptor antagonists on hemodynamics, plasma renin activity, and plasma norepinephrine in hypertension: the key role of vascular resistance changes in relation to partial agonist activity. J Cardiovasc Pharmacol. 1983;5(Suppl 1):S30-45.

7. **Wallin JD, Shah SV.** Beta-adrenergic blocking agents in the treatment of hypertension. Choices based on pharmacological properties and patient characteristics. Arch Intern Med. 1987;147:654-9.

8. **Prisant LM, Mensah GA.** Use of beta-adrenergic receptor blockers in blacks. J Clin Pharmacol. 1996;36:867-73.

9. **Materson BJ, Reda DJ, Cushman WC.** Department of Veterans Affairs Single-Drug therapy of Hypertension Study. Revised figures and new data. Department of Veterans Affairs Cooperative Study Group on Antihypertensive Agents. Am J Hypertens. 1995;8:189-92.

10. **Gibbons RJ, Abrams J, Chatterjee K, et al.** ACC/AHA 2002 guideline update for the management of patients with chronic stable angina—summary article: a report of the American College of Cardiology/American Heart Association Task Force on Practice Guidelines (Committee on the Management of Patients With Chronic Stable Angina). Circulation. 2003;107:149-58.

11. **Hunt SA, Baker DW, Chin MH, et al.** ACC/AHA guidelines for the evaluation and management of chronic heart failure in the adult: executive summary. A report of the American College of Cardiology/American Heart Association Task Force on Practice Guidelines (Committee to revise the 1995 Guidelines for the Evaluation and Management of Heart Failure). J Am Coll Cardiol. 2001;38:2101-13.

12. **Moser M, Prisant LM.** Low-dose combination therapy in hypertension. Am Fam Physician. 1997;56:1275-6,1279,1282.

13. **Ko DT, Hebert PR, Coffey CS, et al.** Beta-blocker therapy and symptoms of depression, fatigue, and sexual dysfunction. JAMA. 2002;288:351-7.

14. **Williams GH.** Converting-enzyme inhibitors in the treatment of hypertension. N Engl J Med. 1988;319:1517-25.

15. **Materson BJ, Preston RA.** Angiotensin-converting enzyme inhibitors in hypertension. A dozen years of experience. Arch Intern Med. 1994;154:513-23.

16. **Arauz-Pacheco C, Parrott MA, Raskin P.** Treatment of hypertension in adults with diabetes. Diabetes Care. 2003;26 Suppl 1:S80-2.

17. **Palmer BF.** Renal dysfunction complicating the treatment of hypertension. N Engl J Med. 2002;347:1256-61.

18. **Goodfriend TL, Elliott ME, Catt KJ.** Angiotensin receptors and their antagonists. N Engl J Med. 1996;334:1649-54.

19. **Burnier M, Brunner HR.** Angiotensin II receptor antagonists. Lancet. 2000;355: 637-45.

20. **Abernethy DR, Schwartz JB.** Calcium-antagonist drugs. N Engl J Med. 1999;341: 1447-57.

21. **Herbette LG, Vecchiarelli M, Sartani A, Leonardi A.** Lercanidipine: short plasma half-life, long duration of action and high cholesterol tolerance. Updated molecular model to rationalize its pharmacokinetic properties. Blood Press Suppl. 1998;2:10-7.

22. **Godfraind T, Salomone S, Dessy C, et al.** Selectivity scale of calcium antagonists in the human cardiovascular system based on in vitro studies. J Cardiovasc Pharmacol. 1992;20(Suppl 5):S34-41.

23. **Prisant L, Elliott W.** Drug delivery systems for treatment of systemic hypertension. Clin Pharmacokinet. 2003;42:931-40.

24. **Psaty BM, Lumley T, Furberg CD, et al.** Health outcomes associated with various antihypertensive therapies used as first-line agents: a network meta-analysis. JAMA. 2003;289:2534-44.

25. **Prisant LM, Herman W.** Calcium channel blocker induced gingival overgrowth. J Clin Hypertens (Greenwich). 2002;4:310-1.

26. **Sica DA, Pool JL.** Alpha-adrenergic blocking drugs: evolving role in clinical medicine. J Clin Hypertens (Greenwich). 2000;2:138-42.

27. **Graham RM, Pettinger WA.** Drug therapy. Prazosin. N Engl J Med. 1979;300:232-6.

28. ALLHAT Collaborative Research Group. Major cardiovascular events in hypertensive patients randomized to doxazosin vs chlorthalidone: The Antihypertensive and Lipid-Lowering Treatment to Prevent Heart Attack Trial (ALLHAT). JAMA. 2000;283: 1967-75.

29. **Neaton JD, Grimm RH, Jr., Prineas RJ, et al.** Treatment of Mild Hypertension Study. Final results. Treatment of Mild Hypertension Study Research Group. JAMA. 1993;270:713-24.

30. **van Zwieten PA.** Centrally acting antihypertensives: a renaissance of interest. Mechanisms and haemodynamics. J Hypertens Suppl. 1997;15:S3-8.

31. **Oster JR, Epstein M.** Use of centrally acting sympatholytic agents in the management of hypertension. Arch Intern Med. 1991;151:1638-44.

32. **Houston MC.** Abrupt cessation of treatment in hypertension: consideration of clinical features, mechanisms, prevention and management of the discontinuation syndrome. Am Heart J. 1981;102(3 Pt 1):415-30.

33. **Woosley RL, Nies AS.** Guanethidine. N Engl J Med. 1976;295:1053-7.

34. **Prisant LM, Spruill WJ, Fincham JE, et al.** Depression associated with antihypertensive drugs. J Fam Pract. 1991;33:481-5.

35. **Koch-Weser J.** Hydralazine. N Engl J Med. 1976;295:320-3.

36. **Pettinger WA.** Minoxidil and the treatment of severe hypertension. N Engl J Med. 1980;303:922-6.

37. Prevention of stroke by antihypertensive drug treatment in older persons with isolated systolic hypertension. Final results of the Systolic Hypertension in the Elderly Program (SHEP). SHEP Cooperative Research Group. JAMA. 1991;265:3255-64.

38. **Staessen JA, Fagard R, Thijs L, et al.** Randomised double-blind comparison of placebo and active treatment for older patients with isolated systolic hypertension. The Systolic Hypertension in Europe (Syst-Eur) Trial Investigators. Lancet. 1997;350:757-64.

39. **Black HR, Elliott WJ, Grandits G, et al.** Principal results of the Controlled Onset Verapamil Investigation of Cardiovascular End Points (CONVINCE) trial. JAMA. 2003;289:2073-82.

40. **Hansson L, Zanchetti A, Carruthers SG, et al.** Effects of intensive blood-pressure lowering and low-dose aspirin in patients with hypertension: principal results of the Hypertension Optimal Treatment (HOT) randomised trial. HOT Study Group. Lancet. 1998;351:1755-62.

7

■ ■ ■

Hypertension and Cardiovascular Disease: Implications of Therapy

Ari Mosenkis, MD

Raymond Townsend, MD

For more than 150 years it has been recognized that elevated systemic arterial pressure is associated with cardiovascular disease. Autopsy studies in the latter half of the 19th century demonstrated structural abnormalities of the heart and kidney that were thought to have been caused by elevated systemic arterial pressure. In 1913, Janeway reported mortalities of 33% from heart failure, 24% from stroke, and 23% from uremia, among 212 hypertensive patients. This was not widely appreciated until 1925 when the Society of Actuaries reported the high mortality of those with hypertension among more than half a million insured men. Since then, the Framingham Heart Study and other investigations have provided longitudinal evidence of the increased risk of cardiovascular disease associated with increasing levels of blood pressure (BP). It has also become clear that hypertension is not a discrete condition, defined by a clear-cut level of BP above which one could be defined as having hypertension and thus at risk for developing these outcomes. Specifically, there is no evidence of any threshold below which lower systolic or diastolic BP is not associated with better outcomes.

In this chapter we review the role of BP in cardiovascular disease with specific coverage of common target organ effects, including renal damage with or without diabetes and with or without proteinuria. We discuss the role of BP in dementia, atrial fibrillation, retinopathy, peripheral arterial disease (PAD), and erectile dysfunction (ED). Lastly we summarize and grade the various classes of antihypertensive medications with respect to their utility in the treatment of hypertension to prevent target organ damage (primary prevention) and in the management of patients who have already sustained a target organ compromise (secondary prevention).

Major Cardiovascular Outcomes

The major cardiovascular outcomes of hypertension are stroke, myocardial infarction, congestive heart failure (CHF), and end-stage renal disease (ESRD) (Table 7-1). These outcomes are significant because of their large associated morbidity and mortality, as well as the strong evidence implicating hypertension as an independent risk factor for these conditions. Other cardiovascular outcomes with less significant morbidity and mortality and/or weaker associations with BP are summarized in Table 7-2.

All Cardiovascular Outcomes

Abundant evidence proves that control of BP improves cardiovascular outcomes (see Chapter 3). The Veterans Administration Cooperative Study was the first large, prospective, placebo-controlled trial to document significant reductions in certain cardiovascular events (stroke and heart failure) with the use of available antihypertensive agents in essential hypertension. Since then, hundreds of medication trials, meta-analyses, and consensus reports have been published. A meta-analysis by Moser and Herbert of 20 early antihypertensive trials documented the impressive impact of antihypertensive therapy on cardiovascular outcomes, as shown in Figure 7-1 (1). All of the earlier studies used diuretic or beta-blocker–based regimens. When compared

Table 7-1   Cardiovascular Outcomes of Hypertension

Major Cardiovascular Outcomes	Other Cardiovascular Outcomes
• Stroke	• Dementia
• Myocardial infarction	• Atrial fibrillation
• Congestive heart failure	• Retinopathy
• End-stage renal disease	• Peripheral arterial disease
	• Erectile dysfunction

Table 7-2   Risk Factors for the Progression of Hypertensive Nephrosclerosis to End-Stage Renal Disease

• Presence of concurrent renal insufficiency of another etiology

• Proteinuria

• Diabetes mellitus

• Black race

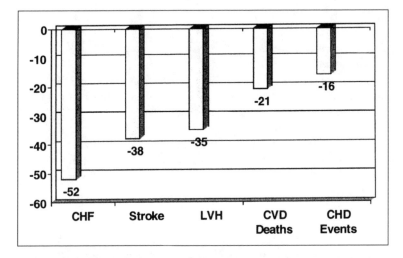

Figure 7-1 Relative-risk reductions of selected cardiovascular outcomes based on a meta-analysis of 20 early diuretic and beta-blocker based antihypertensive trials.

with beta-blockers, diuretics have generally been more effective at both lowering BP and preventing cardiovascular outcomes. Consequently, diuretics have traditionally been recommended as first-line antihypertensive therapy. With the introduction of angiotensin-converting enzyme (ACE) inhibitors, some controversy arose regarding which agent is the most effective in preventing all outcomes. Two recent studies, one a placebo-controlled study and the other a randomized comparison of ACE inhibitors to diuretics, have fueled this controversy. The first such study was the Heart Outcomes Prevention Evaluation Study (HOPE), which showed that ramipril, versus placebo, significantly decreased all cardiovascular outcomes, although only half of the subjects enrolled in the HOPE trial had hypertension, and only a small part of the benefit could be attributed to a reduction in BP (2).

The other report was the Second Australian National Blood Pressure Study (ANBP2). It reported a better reduction of all cardiovascular outcomes with the use of an ACE inhibitor versus a diuretic, despite similar reductions in BP (3). Notably, in a subgroup analysis this effect was only statistically significant in male subjects. Conversely, the Antihypertensive and Lipid-Lowering Treatment to Prevent Heart Attack Trial (ALLHAT) clearly demonstrated that thiazide-type diuretics are as effective as calcium channel blockers or ACE inhibitors in preventing any cardiovascular outcome (4). Consequently, based on the established record of endpoint reduction and the widespread availability of cheap generic products, the recently published Seventh Report of the Joint National Committee on Prevention, Detection, Evaluation and Treatment of High Blood Pressure (JNC-7) recommended thiazide-type diuretics as the first-line therapy for hypertension in the absence of other compelling indication (5).

Stroke

Hypertension as a Risk Factor for Stroke

The Framingham Heart Study confirmed the role of hypertension as a risk factor for stroke. Further epidemiological data from the Framingham Study has shown a continuous, linear relationship between BP and the incidence of stroke. More recent data has shown that elevated systolic BP, as opposed to diastolic BP, is the predominant risk factor for stroke in elderly subjects (in whom most strokes occur). A recent meta-analysis of eight trials assessing outcomes in isolated systolic hypertension in the elderly found that each 10 mm Hg increase in initial systolic BP above 160 increased stroke risk by 22% (6).

Effect of Control of Hypertension in Lowering Stroke Risk

Many randomized, prospective, placebo-controlled trials have documented the benefit of BP lowering in stroke prevention. Notably, the Systolic Hypertension in the Elderly Program (SHEP) demonstrated a 36% reduction in incidence of stroke in older subjects with the use of low doses of the thiazide-like diuretic chlorthalidone, as depicted in Figure 7-2. The Systolic Hypertension in Europe (Syst-Eur) trial demonstrated a 44% reduction in the incidence of stroke with the use of nitrendipine-based therapy (7). Thus, stroke is the cardiovascular outcome upon which control of hypertension has the largest impact. More recently, a large meta-analysis has suggested that calcium channel blockers are more effective than diuretics or beta-blockers in preventing stroke (8). This meta-analysis was completed before the ALLHAT data became available. ALLHAT found that chlorthalidone was equivalent to amlodipine but superior to lisinopril (in blacks, non-diabetics, and women) in preventing stroke. In the presence of left ventricular hypertrophy (LVH), angiotensin-receptor blockers (ARBs), when compared with beta-blockers, are particularly effective at stroke prevention, as shown in the Losartan Intervention for Endpoint reduction in hypertension (LIFE) study (9).

Regarding the prevention of recurrent stroke, the data published by the Perindopril Protection Against Recurrent Stroke Study (PROGRESS) Collaborative Group support the use of a combination of an ACE inhibitor and a diuretic (10). Consequently, although the JNC-7 report recommends a diuretic for prevention of first stroke, it recommends a combination of ACE inhibitor and diuretic as therapy for prevention of recurrent stroke.

Coronary Artery Disease and Myocardial Infarction

Hypertension as a Risk Factor for Coronary Heart Disease

Hypertension is a strong, independent risk factor for ischemic heart disease, the most common major cardiovascular outcome associated with hypertension. In the Multiple Risk Factor Intervention Trial (MRFIT), heart attacks were twice as common in those with a screening diastolic BP of >90 among

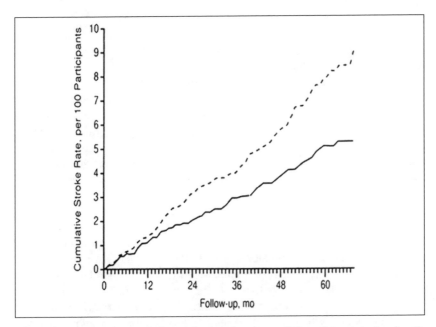

Figure 7-2 Cumulative fatal plus nonfatal stroke rate per 100 participants in the diuretic arm (*solid line*) and placebo arm (*broken line*) during the Systolic Hypertension in the Elderly Program. (Courtesy of SHEP Cooperative Research Group, Prevention of stroke by antihypertensive drug treatment in older persons with isolated systolic hypertension. Final results of the Systolic Hypertension in the Elderly Program (SHEP). JAMA. 1991;265:3255-64. Copyright 1991, American Medical Association. All rights reserved; with permission.)

more than 325,000 men (11). As is the case with stroke, the Framingham data show a graded, linear association between BP and myocardial infarction.

Effect of Control of Hypertension in Lowering Risk for Coronary Heart Disease

Multiple studies have shown that sucessful management of hypertension can reduce coronary heart disease risk, although such effect is less impressive than that for stroke prevention. For example, prospective studies demonstrate that a reduction of 5-6 mm Hg in diastolic BP is associated with a 35%-40% reduction in the incidence of stroke but only a 20%-25% reduction in the incidence of coronary heart disease. This is likely the case because stroke is associated with hypertension more than any other risk factor, whereas coronary disease is more a function of atherosclerosis, which is influenced by other factors (e.g., lipids, smoking, and diabetes) as much as by hypertension.

No one agent has been shown to be superior in preventing coronary heart disease, but evidence supports the use of beta-blockers to prevent myocardial infarction in patients with known coronary heart disease. Additionally, beta-blockers, ACE inhibitors, and aldosterone antagonists are all recommended by JNC-7 for patients post–myocardial infarction.

Congestive Heart Failure

Hypertension as a Risk Factor for Development of Congestive Heart Failure

The impact of hypertension on CHF is difficult to document without long-term follow-up because it is a later manifestation of hypertension. Hypertensive patients initially develop LVH and progress to systolic dysfunction after prolonged exposure to elevated left ventricular pressure (afterload). Thus, in one large study of hypertensive patients CHF was a rare occurrence before 10 years (incidence <1 per 1000 patient years), but the incidence rose sharply (to nearly 3 per 1000 patient years) thereafter (Figure 7-3).

Effect of Control of Hypertension in Lowering Risk of Congestive Heart Failure

Evidence clearly demonstrates that control of BP lowers the incidence of CHF. In the meta-analysis by Moser and Herbert of 20 early studies using diuretic and beta-blocker-based regimens (Figure 7-1), the relative risk reduction for primary prevention of CHF and LVH were 52% and 35%, respectively (1). Again, some controversy arose regarding the use of ACE inhibitors as primary prevention for this outcome. When all available data were reviewed in a large meta-analysis, low-dose diuretics were shown to be more effective than ACE inhibitors, beta-blockers, or calcium channel blockers at preventing this outcome. Likewise, ALLHAT found diuretics more effective than ACE inhibitors, calcium channel blockers, or alpha blockers in CHF prevention.

On the other hand, in patients with LVH and in those with established CHF, thiazide diuretics might not be the first choice. ACE inhibitors and ARBs

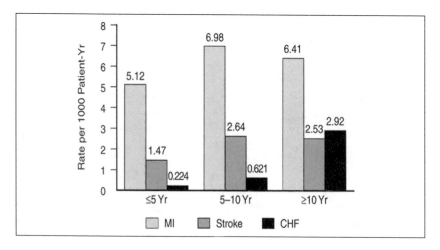

Figure 7-3   Changing patterns of cardiovascular events according to time in therapy. (From Hypertension: A Companion to Brenner and Rector's The Kidney. Oparil S and Weber MA, eds. Philadelphia: WB Saunders; 2000: 225; with permission.)

have been shown to be most effective in causing regression of LVH, although any agent other than the direct vasodilators (hydralazine and minoxidil) will work to a lesser degree. The previously cited LIFE study confirms support for the morbidity and mortality benefits of angiotensin-receptor blockade in patients with LVH.

Specific Agents That Decrease Mortality in Patients with Congestive Heart Failure

In patients with systolic dysfunction (many of whom no longer have elevated BP) numerous trials, including the Studies of Left Ventricular Dysfunction trial (SOLVD), the Cooperative North Scandinavian Enalapril Survival Study (CONSENSUS), and others, have documented the benefits of ACE inhibitors in decreasing mortality. Similarly, the Valsartan Heart Failure Trial (ValHeFT) has demonstrated the benefits of ARBs in decreasing mortality. The beta-blockers carvedilol and metoprolol, and the mineralocorticoid-receptor antagonist (MRA) spironolactone have also been shown to significantly decrease mortality in those with CHF. These effects are generally thought to occur independently of lowering BP. Though thiazide-type diuretics are the most effective agents in preventing the onset of CHF, no randomized controlled trial has looked at the impact of diuretics (thiazide or loop) on mortality in people already diagnosed with CHF. Nevertheless, diuretics (primary loop diuretics) are essential components in the management of patients with CHF, along with digoxin, ACE inhibitors (or ARBs), and MRAs.

End-Stage Renal Disease

Hypertension as a Risk Factor for Development of Renal Failure

Malignant hypertension has long been recognized as a risk factor for the development of renal failure. It had been unclear, however, whether mild elevations of BP increase the risk of developing ESRD. In 1996, the MRFIT trial clearly demonstrated a positive graded relationship between systolic and diastolic BP and the incidence of ESRD among 332,544 men (Figures 7-4 and 7-5) (12). This and other studies have thus helped clarify the risk factors for the progression of hypertensive nephrosclerosis to ESRD, as summarized in Table 7-2.

Effect of Control of Hypertension in Delaying Progression of Non-Diabetic Renal Failure

Multiple studies have shown the benefit of treating hypertension in delaying the progression of hypertensive or other non-diabetic chronic kidney disease (CKD) to ESRD. Specifically, the Modification of Diet in Renal Disease (MDRD) trial, which excluded patients with insulin-dependent diabetes, demonstrated that tight control of BP is effective in slowing the progression of CKD, although this was evident only in those with significant proteinuria (13). The recently published meta-analysis by Jafar et al demonstrated that

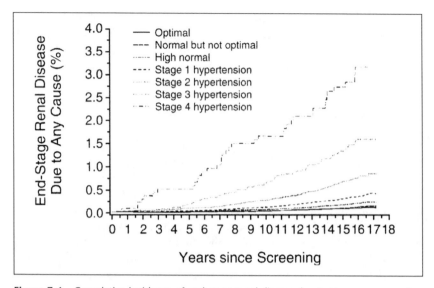

Figure 7-4 Cumulative incidence of end-stage renal disease due to any cause according to blood-pressure category in 332,544 men screened for MRFIT. Stages of blood pressure were taken from JNC-5. (From Klag MJ, Whelton PK, Randall BL, et al. Blood pressure and end-stage renal disease in men. N Engl J Med. 1996;334:13-8; with permission.)

among non-diabetics with CKD, greater protein excretion and systolic (but not diastolic) BP levels were independently related to increased risk for worsening kidney disease (14). They also found that systolic BP less than 110 mm Hg may be associated with a higher risk for kidney disease progression, although this phenomenon is likely in part due to underlying poor health in patients with the lowest BPs. Jafar et al recommended a systolic BP goal between 110 and 129 mm Hg in patients with greater than 1 gram/day of urinary protein excretion.

ACE inhibitors have been shown to be particularly beneficial in preserving renal function in non-diabetic patients with CKD. The ACE-Inhibition in Progressive Renal Insufficiency (AIPRI) Study Group showed that benazepril versus placebo offers a 53% risk reduction of renal endpoints (doubling of serum creatinine or need for dialysis) among non-diabetics with CKD, more than 80% of whom had hypertension. Other drugs that may be used are shown in Table 7-3.

Effect of Control of Hypertension in Delaying Progression of Diabetic Renal Failure

A considerable body of evidence shows that inhibition of the renin-angiotensin system is exceptionally useful in delaying the progression of CKD in patients with diabetic nephropathy. The Collaborative Study Group demonstrated the utility of ACE inhibitors in proteinuric type-I diabetics, and a similar benefit has been demonstrated with the use of the ARBs losartan and

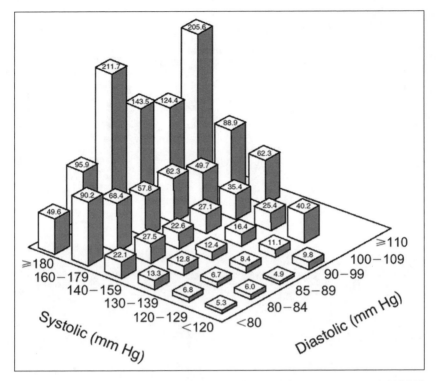

Figure 7-5   Age-adjusted rate of end-stage renal disease due to any cause per 100,000 person-years, according to systolic and diastolic blood pressure in 332,544 men screened for MRFIT. (From Klag MJ, Whelton PK, Randall BL, et al. Blood pressure and end-stage renal disease in men. N Engl J Med. 1996;334:13-8; with permission.)

irbesartan in patients with type-II diabetes (15). Thus, in both diabetic and non-diabetic patients with proteinuric renal failure, the recommendation is to lower the urinary protein excretion using ACE inhibitors or ARBs (or a combination) as the agents of first choice. There are sparse data showing any benefit of lowering proteinuria to less than 1 gram/day, but it is reasonable to increase doses of ACE inhibitors and ARBs as tolerated to lower the degree of proteinuria as much as possible, especially in patients with diabetic nephropathy. Other drugs options to be used adjunctively with ACE inhibitors and/or ARBs are shown in Table 7-3. The pharmacologic treatment of hypertension associated with renal disease is discussed in greater detail in Chapter 8.

Tight Blood Pressure Control in Patients with Non-Proteinuric Renal Failure

Controversy remains regarding the role of aggressive BP control in patients with CKD and minimal proteinuria. In the MDRD trial, the AIPRI study, and the meta-analysis by Jafar et al, tight BP control in patients with less than 1 to 2 grams/day of urinary protein excretion was not significantly associated

Table 7-3   Efficacy of Antihypertensive Agent Classes for Selected Cardiovascular Outcomes

	Diuretic	Beta Blocker	Non-dihydropyridine CCB	Dihydropyridine CCB	ACE Inhibitor	ARB	MRB
Prevent first stroke	Superior	Effective	Effective	Superior	Effective	Superior in LVH patients	—
Prevent recurrent stroke	Superior	Effective		Effective	Superior	—	—
Prevent MI (first or recurrent) in CAD patients	—	Effective	—	—	Effective	—	Effective
Lower mortality in CHD patients	Essential	Effective	—	—	Effective	Effective	Effective
LVH regression	—	Effective	—	—	Superior	Superior	—
Delay progression of CKD in nondiabetics	Effective	Effective	—	—	Superior	Effective	—
Delay progression of CKD in type I diabetics	Effective	Effective	Effective	—	Superior	Effective	—
Delay progression of CKD in type II diabetics	—	—	Effective; used adjunctively with ACE inhibitors or ARBs	—	Essential	Superior	—
Prevent dementia	—	—	—	Effective	—	—	—
Prevent post-MI or post-cardioversion atrial fibrillation	—	—	—	—	Effective	Effective	—
Regression of grade III or IV hypertensive retinopathy	Effective	Effective	—	—	—	—	—
Regression of diabetic retinopathy	—	Effective	—	—	Effective	—	—
Ameliorate claudication in PAD patients	—	—	Effective	—	—	—	—
Prevent all cardiovascular end-points in high-risk patients	Superior	—	—	—	Superior	—	—

CCB = calcium channel blocker; ACE = angiotensin-converting enzyme; ARB = angiotensin-receptor blocker; MRB = mineralocorticoid-receptor blocker.

with a lower risk of progression of CKD. These conclusions are similar to those of the African American Study of Kidney Disease and Hypertension Study Group (AASK). The AASK study randomized African-American subjects with hypertensive renal disease, excluding subjects with diabetes or with greater than 2.5 grams/day of proteinuria, to a lower or a usual BP goal. They observed no additional benefit of tight BP control in slowing the progression of renal failure.

More careful analysis of the MDRD data reveals that in the group of patients with baseline moderate proteinuria (1-3 grams/day) a benefit can be demonstrated after prolonged follow-up (more than 24 months) as demonstrated in Figure 7-6. The explanation for this phenomenon is as follows:

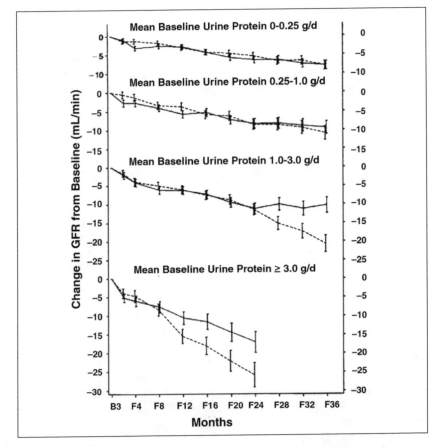

Figure 7-6 Estimated mean decline in glomerular filtration rate stratified by four quartiles of baseline proteinuria. The usual (*dashed lines*) and low (*solid lines*) are compared. B3 equals the third monthly baseline visit (before randomization); F equals follow-up visits at each given number of months. (From Peterson JC, Adler S, Burkart JM, et al. Blood pressure control, proteinuria, and the progression of renal disease. The Modification of Diet in Renal Disease Study. Ann Intern Med. 1995;123:754-62; with permission.).

Proteinuria is both nephrotoxic and a marker for severity of kidney disease. Thus, proteinuric conditions tend to progress to ESRD more quickly while forms of CKD with lower levels of proteinuria progress more slowly. Consequently, as was illustrated above by CHF, it is difficult to demonstrate the efficacy of any intervention in patients with CKD and low levels of proteinuria without studying large numbers of subjects for a prolonged period of time. Thus, JNC-7 recommends a target BP of less than 130/80 for all patients with CKD (defined as a GFR <60 mL/min/1.73m^2 or albuminuria >300 mg/day).

Furthermore, even if aggressive BP control has a limited impact on renal outcomes in patients with low levels of proteinuria, one should not conclude that such control is of no benefit. On the contrary, patients with CKD are considered to be in the highest risk category for suffering major cardiovascular outcomes such as stroke, myocardial infarction, and the development of CHF; the desire to prevent these outcomes mandates good BP control, preferably including ACE inhibition as recommended by the authors of the HOPE study. The negative results of MDRD, AIPRI, AASK, etc. only highlight the reality that current therapies, even as they delay or prevent other major cardiovascular outcomes, are not particularly effective in preventing renal outcomes in patients with low levels of proteinuria.

Other Cardiovascular Outcomes

Dementia

Hypertension as a Potential Risk Factor for the Development of Dementia

The observation that strokes often cause cognitive decline has led many to speculate that hypertension might itself be a risk factor for the development of dementia. The evidence, however, is inconsistent. Specifically, an analysis of 1702 stroke-free Framingham Study participants found an inverse relationship between systolic and diastolic BPs taken in the 1950s and 1960s and the subsequent scoring 20 years later on tests to measure cognitive function (15). Likewise, the Honolulu-Asia Aging Study found a significant relationship between systolic BP (but not diastolic BP) at enrollment and the risk of cognitive impairment 25 years later (16). Some controversy exists, however, and several studies were unable to document this association. Other groups have even shown a positive association between BP and cognitive function.

The inconsistency of data likely stems from the notion that, similar to CHF, dementia is a late manifestation of hypertension, and the effects of BP on cognitive function can be best studied only with very long follow-up. Additionally, data show that BPs measured within a few years of the development of dementia positively correlate with cognitive function. These results suggest that although hypertension is a risk factor for the development of dementia several decades later, it is associated with higher cognitive function in the short term. It is unclear whether this association exists because higher BP provides better perfusion of the brain or because patients with higher cognitive function exhibit more physical activity, which is associated with higher BP. Alternatively, a diseased brain may be less able to provide the "autonomic output" necessary for the maintenance of high BP. Moreover, the use of different tools for assessing cognition, even when testing a single cohort, has yielded disparate results.

Prevention of Dementia Through Hypertension Control

The notion that hypertension is a risk factor for the development of dementia has generated great interest in investigating the effects of anti-hypertensive therapy on the subsequent decline of cognitive function. Several prospective observational studies have documented a lower incidence of dementia in elderly hypertensive patients whose BP were treated pharmacologically compared with those who were not treated. Subsequently, several groups tested this hypothesis using data from prospective, randomized, placebo-controlled trials. Surprisingly, both the SHEP study and the Medical Research Council trial failed to demonstrate a significant effect of treatment of hypertension on the incidence of dementia. The Syst-Eur trial demonstrated that treatment with nitrendipine (a dihydropyridine calcium antagonist) reduced the incidence of dementia by 55% (Figure 7-7) (17).

These results have been questioned because large numbers of patients were lost to follow-up. Furthermore, some have suggested that the positive association was attributable to calcium channel antagonism, irrespective of the effect on BP. The Study on Cognition and Prognosis in the Elderly (SCOPE) trial recently reported that the ARB candesartan was no more effective than placebo in preventing the onset of dementia among nearly 5000 elderly hypertensive patients (18). One explanation for the lack of a strong effect of BP control on the incidence of dementia is that, as stated above, dementia is a very late cardiovascular outcome. Research to assess the true impact of anti-hypertensive therapy needs to be conducted in large groups of patients with very long follow-up.

Atrial Fibrillation

Hypertension as a Risk Factor for Developing Atrial Fibrillation

Data from the Framingham Study revealed that the risk of developing atrial fibrillation in hypertensive subjects is nearly twice the risk in normotensive controls (19). Subgroup analysis of these results shows that the risk is greatest in those with radiographic or electrocardiographic evidence of cardiomegaly. In the absence of such findings, the association is weak. The Manitoba Follow-Up Study followed nearly 4000 recruits in the Royal

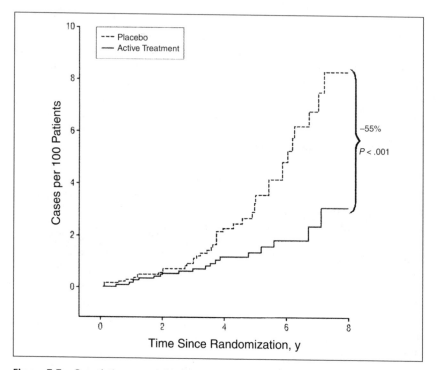

Figure 7-7 Cumulative rate of dementia in the nitrendipine arm (*solid line*) and placebo arm (*dotted line*) in the Syst-Eur study. (From Forette F, Seux ML, Staessen JA, et al. Systolic Hypertension in Europe Investigators. The prevention of dementia with antihypertensive treatment: new evidence from the Systolic Hypertension in Europe (Syst-Eur) study. Arch Intern Med. 2002;162:2046-52; with permission.

Canadian Air Force and found the relative risk of developing atrial fibrillation among those with hypertension to be 2.3 (20). This risk dropped to 1.4 when adjusted in a multivariate Cox model. Despite this relatively weak association, hypertension, because of its high prevalence, is still the most common recognized comorbidity in patients with atrial fibrillation.

Antihypertensive Therapy for Prevention of Atrial Fibrillation

Antihypertensive therapy has been shown to lead to regression of structural changes in the heart associated with atrial fibrillation such as atrial enlargement and LVH. Consequently, antihypertensive therapy should, in theory, reduce the incidence of new or recurrent atrial fibrillation (21). The evidence to support this notion, however, is sparse. Specifically, an ACE inhibitor has been shown to reduce the incidence of atrial fibrillation after acute myocardial infarction, and an ARB has been shown to maintain sinus rhythm after cardioversion in patients with atrial fibrillation. These results were independent of any change in BP, and are likely attributable to blockade of the renin-angiotensin system.

Retinopathy

Clinical Significance of Hypertensive Retinopathy

In 1850, Hermann von Helmholtz invented the ophthalmoscope. Nine years later Liebreich was the first to describe abnormalities of the retina in a patient with probable hypertension. The prevalence of hypertensive retinopathy has only recently been described. The Beaver Dam Eye Study and the Blue Mountains Eye Study have reported a prevalence of retinopathy of 8% to 10% among non-diabetic hypertensive patients. The incidence increases with age and with severity (or poor control) of hypertension.

The clinical significance of hypertensive retinopathy was not apparent until 1939 when a group of physicians at the Mayo Clinic classified hypertensive patients based on the severity of retinal disease and showed that those with more severe disease had higher morbidity and mortality. Although there are numerous case reports of hypertensive retinopathy progressing to blindness, either directly (via retinal infarction, retinal hemorrhage, disc edema, or vitreous hemorrhage) or indirectly (via infarction of the visual cortex or optic nerve, occlusion of retinal vessels, or raised intracranial BP), hypertensive retinopathy is not a major cause of blindness. Most of the case reports are in patients with severe malignant hypertension, including those whose BPs were lowered too rapidly. Thus, hypertensive retinopathy should be viewed more as a marker for other major cardiovascular outcomes, particularly microvascular outcomes such as renal insufficiency.

Effect of Control of Hypertension in Ameliorating Retinopathy

The assessment of changes in eye-ground characteristics during antihypertensive treatment is not a common feature of clinical trials in hypertension. Nevertheless, several older studies attest to the ability of BP reduction with diuretics and beta-blockers, particularly from severely elevated levels, to result in improvement in hypertensive retinopathy. In general, grade III and IV retinopathy will improve with good BP control achieved with any antihypertensive regimen. Grade I and II retinopathy are more general in origin, occurring in association with other factors such as aging and atherosclerosis, and do not necessarily improve with antihypertensive therapy; nor is their persistence necessarily a sign of inadequate treatment.

Hypertension as a Risk Factor for Progression of Diabetic Retinopathy

Hypertension is a major risk factor for the progression of diabetic retinopathy, which is the leading cause of blindness in the United States and affects more than 5 million adults. The association between hypertension and diabetic retinopathy has been demonstrated by numerous studies including the Atherosclerosis Risk in Communities Study (ARIC), the United Kingdom Prospective Diabetes Study Group (UKPDS), and the Appropriate Blood Pressure Control in Diabetes Trial (ABCD).

Tight BP Control as Prevention of Diabetic Retinopathy Progession
There exists some controversy regarding the impact of tight control of BP
on the progression of diabetic retinopathy. The UKPDS study showed that
among patients with type II diabetes followed for 9 years tight BP control
(144/82 mm Hg compared with 154/87 mm Hg) achieved a 47% reduction of
the risk of progression of diabetic retinopathy (22). No difference in outcome
was noted between the use of an ACE inhibitor or a beta-blocker. On the
other hand, the ABCD trial found no statistically significant difference between intensive (132/78 mm Hg) and moderate BP control (138/86 mm Hg)
over 5 years of follow-up. Furthermore, no difference was found between
use of an ACE inhibitor and a dihydropyridine calcium channel blocker.

The discrepancy between the two studies is likely related to several factors. First, the BP levels achieved in the ABCD trial were far better than
those achieved in the UKPDS. Specifically, the moderate control group in
the ABCD trial had lower systolic BPs (138/86 mm Hg) than the tight control
arm of the UKPDS (144/82 mm Hg) Furthermore, the UKPDS was a large
study (1148 patients) with largely disparate BP goals. The ABCD trial was
smaller (470 patients) and had BP targets that were much less disparate.
Finally, the UKPDS followed its patients for nearly twice the duration of the
ABCD trial. Thus, it appears that BP control does significantly reduce the
risk of progression of diabetic retinopathy. It is unclear, however, if this
effect levels off once the BP is only moderately controlled, with little additional benefit incurred by more aggressive control. Furthermore, the consequences are best observed after long-term follow-up.

Several studies have specifically investigated the effects of ACE inhibition
on the progression of diabetic retinopathy in normotensive type I and type 2
diabetics. Three prospective trials from the early 1990s failed to show a benefit of ACE inhibitors, possibly because of insufficient power. A later trial
(and meta-analysis) did demonstrate a protective effect of lisinopril on diabetic retinopathy in normotensive subjects, although the results have been
questioned because of better glycemic control in the lisinopril arm (23).

Peripheral Arterial Disease

Hypertension as a Risk Factor for Peripheral Arterial Disease
PAD is a common condition that is strongly and independently associated
with hypertension. Data from the Framingham study demonstrate a graded
relationship between BP and the risk of intermittent claudication (a surrogate for PAD), with an odds ratio of 1.3 for "high-normal" BP (130-139/85-
89), 1.5 for "Stage 1" hypertension (140-159/90-99), and 2.2 for "Stage 2"
hypertension (>160/>100) as defined by JNC-6 criteria (Figure 7-8).

Control of Hypertension to Prevent or Delay Peripheral Arterial Disease
Although it is reasonable to assume that adequate control of BP would prevent or delay the onset of PAD, there are only sparse data to support this

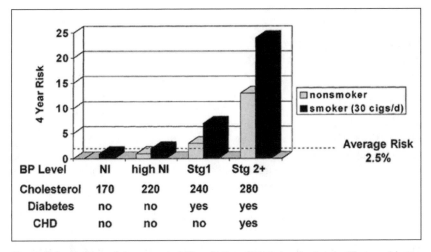

Figure 7-8   Estimated 4-year probability of intermittent claudication in 70-year-old men in the Framingham Heart Study. Stg 1, stage 1 hypertension; Stg 2+, stage 2 or greater hypertension; CHD, coronary heart disease; cigs, cigarettes. (From Murabito JM, D'Agostino RB, Silbershatz H, Wilson PW. Intermittent claudication: a risk profile from the Framingham Heart Study. Circulation. 1997;96:44-9; with permission.)

notion. Nor is there any existing evidence that antihypertensive therapy alters the progression of PAD, once established. Verapamil has been shown to be effective in ameliorating the symptoms of intermittent claudication, although the effect is related to the vasodilatory effects of calcium antagonism and is independent of any lowering of BP. Nevertheless, PAD is a strong risk factor for other cardiovascular outcomes, such as stroke and myocardial infarction. Thus, aggressive control of hypertension is warranted to prevent these outcomes, even if the effects vis-à-vis progression of PAD are negligible.

JNC-7 makes no specific recommendation in terms of which antihypertensive medication to use in hypertensive individuals with this condition. There exists some controversy, however, regarding the use of beta-blockers. Beta-blockers were once considered relatively contraindicated in patients with PAD because of the perception that these agents could worsen the symptoms of claudication. This misconception has been dispelled by multiple prospective, randomized, placebo-controlled trials and a meta-analysis. One report found that neither atenolol nor the dihydropyridine calcium channel blocker, nifedipine, had any adverse or beneficial effects on claudication symptoms when used alone. However, the combination of the two agents adversely affected walking ability, without any relation to change in BP. Thus, it would be prudent to avoid this combination. An ACE inhibitor or a diuretic would be the agent of first choice, based on the conclusions of the HOPE trial and ALLHAT study, respectively, in patients with high cardiovascular risk.

Erectile Dysfunction

Hypertension as a Risk Factor for Erectile Dysfunction

Erectile dysfunction, also known as (one form of) male sexual dysfunction, or impotence, has long been observed to be prevalent among men with high BP. Though some controversy exists, most of the larger reports (including the Massachusetts Male Aging Study and numerous large cross-sectional studies in the United States and Europe) have supported this observation. Additionally, ED has been found to be more severe among subjects with hypertension. The reported odds ratios and relative risks range from 1.13 to 1.89, with treated hypertension typically exhibiting a stronger association because antihypertensive therapy is itself associated with ED.

Treatment of Hypertension Does Not Ameliorate Symptoms of Erectile Dysfunction

There are no long-term data to assess whether early treatment of hypertension can prevent the onset of ED. Rather, ED is listed as a side effect of virtually all antihypertensive agents (although, with the possible exception of some beta-blockers, the incidence of ED reported with antihypertensive agents is probably not significantly higher than the incidence reported with placebo). It is not clear whether ED is a specific drug effect or if it is simply a response to the lowering of systemic arterial pressure.

Importance of Questioning Hypertensive Men About Erectile Dysfunction

When treating men for hypertension it is important both to ask them about the presence of ED and to warn them about its potential occurrence. ED is associated with a poorer quality of life. Furthermore, if perceived to be an adverse effect of a medication, the likelihood of non-adherence with the regimen significantly increases. Thus, the development of ED after the initiation of a particular antihypertensive agent would mandate switching to a different drug class, even if that drug-class is less indicated for any specific outcome. Additionally, as mentioned above with respect to some kidney diseases, retinopathy, and PAD, ED can be viewed as a marker for other cardiovascular outcomes. Therefore, if ED is present, one might choose to be more aggressive about controlling other risk factors such as smoking, high cholesterol, and diabetes.

Summary

Hypertension represents an objectively measured and reproducible cardiovascular risk factor. Control of hypertension generally reduces risk of target organ compromise, with some classes of antihypertensive agents performing better than others. This may be due to superior BP reduction achieved with the use of that agent class, or it may be the result of more specific (or more complete) interruption of pathophysiologic cascades such as the renin-angiotensin system.

■ ■ ■

Key Points

- The major cardiovascular outcomes of hypertension are stroke, myocardial infarction, congestive heart failure, and end-stage renal disease; all four have significant associated morbidity and mortality, and there is strong evidence implicating hypertension as an independent risk factor in these conditions.

- JNC-7 recommends thiazide-type diuretics as first-line therapy for hypertension in the absence of another compelling indication.

- Stroke is the cardiovascular outcome upon which control of hypertension has the largest impact. Large placebo-controlled antihypertensive trials have demonstrated a 36%-44% reduction in incidence of stroke.

- Ischemic heart disease is the most common major cardiovascular outcome associated with hypertension. The impact of BP control on ischemic heart disease is less marked than it is on stroke, but it has an absolute risk reduction of 20%-25%. Thus, other risk factors for atherosclerosis must be addressed in hypertensive patients.

- The impact of hypertension on CHF is difficult to document without long-term follow-up because CHF is a later manifestation of hypertension.

- In diabetic and non-diabetic patients with proteinuric renal failure, blockade of the renin-angiotensin system with an ACE inhibitor or an ARB to lower BP and to decrease proteinuria to less than 2 grams/day will reduce the risk of progression to ESRD.

- In patients with less than 1-2 grams/day of proteinuria, it likely that further renal protection is offered by more aggressive BP control. Such control is also critical to prevent other cardiovascular outcomes.

- Hypertension is a risk factor for the development of dementia several decades after onset, although it is associated with higher cognitive function in the short term.

- Hypertensive retinopathy it not a major cause of blindness; however, it should be viewed as a marker for other major cardiovascular outcomes, particularly microvascular outcomes such as renal insufficiency. Hypertension is, nonetheless, a major risk factor for progression of diabetic retinopathy, although it is unclear whether aggressive control offers more benefit than moderate control in preventing blindness.

- Although hypertension is a risk factor for development of peripheral artery disease, there are only sparse data to support the notion that antihypertensive therapy can alter progression of PAD once it is present. Nevertheless, similar to non-proteinuric chronic kidney disease and hypertensive retinopathy, aggressive control of hypertension is warranted to prevent other major cardiovascular outcomes.

■   ■   ■

REFERENCES

1. **Moser M, Hebert PR.** Prevention of disease progression, left ventricular hypertrophy and CHF in hypertension treatment trials. J Am Coll Cardiol. 1996;27:1214-8.

2. **Yusuf S, Sleight P, Pogue J, et al.** Effects of an angiotensin-converting enzyme inhibitor, ramipril, on cardiovascular events in high-risk patients. N Engl J Med. 2000;342:145-53.

3. **Wing LM, Reid CM, Ryan P, et al.** Second Australian National Blood Pressure Study Group. A comparison of outcomes with angiotensin-converting enzyme inhibitors and diuretics for hypertension in the elderly. N Engl J Med. 2003;348:583-92.

4. ALLHAT Officers and Coordinators for the ALLHAT Collaborative Research Group. The Antihypertensive and Lipid-Lowering Treatment to Prevent Heart Attack Trial. Major outcomes in high-risk hypertensive patients randomized to angiotensin-converting enzyme inhibitor or calcium channel blocker vs diuretic: the Antihypertensive and Lipid-Lowering Treatment to Prevent Heart Attack Trial (ALLHAT). JAMA. 2002;288:2981-97.

5. **Chobanian AV, Bakris GL, Black HR, et al.** The Seventh Report of the Joint National Committee on Prevention, Detection, Evaluation and Treatment of High Blood Pressure. JAMA. 2003;289:2560-72.

6. **Staessen JA, Gasowski J, Wang JG, et al.** Risks of untreated and treated isolated systolic hypertension in the elderly: meta-analysis of outcome trials. Lancet. 2000;355:865-72.

7. **Staessen JA, Fagard R, Thijs L, et al.** Randomised double-blind comparison of placebo and active treatment for older patients with isolated systolic hypertension. The Systolic Hypertension in Europe (Syst-Eur) Trial Investigators. Lancet. 1997;350:757-64.

8. **Neal B, MacMahon S, Chapman N.** Blood Pressure Lowering Treatment Trialists' Collaboration. Effects of ACE inhibitors, calcium antagonists, and other blood-pressure-lowering drugs: results of prospectively designed overviews of randomized trials. Lancet. 2000;356:1955-64.

9. **Dahlof B, Devereux RB, Kjeldsen SE, et al.** LIFE Study Group. Cardiovascular morbidity and mortality in the Losartan Intervention for Endpoint Reduction in Hypertension Study (LIFE): a randomised trial against atenolol. Lancet. 2002;359:995-1003.

10. PROGRESS Collaborative Group. Randomized trial of a perindopril-based blood-pressure-lowering regimen among 6105 individuals with previous stroke or transient ischaemic attack. Lancet. 2001;358:1033-41.

11. **Kannel WB, Neaton JD, Wentworth D, et al.** Overall and coronary heart disease mortality rates in relation to major risk factors in 325,348 men screened for the MRFIT. Multiple Risk Factor Intervention Trial. Am Heart J. 1986;112:825-36.

12. **Klag MJ, Whelton PK, Randall BL, et al.** Blood pressure and end-stage renal disease in men. N Engl J Med. 1996;334:13-8.

13. **Klahr S, Levey AS, Beck GJ, et al.** The effects of dietary protein restriction and blood-pressure control on the progression of chronic renal disease. New Engl J Med. 1994;330:877-84.

14. **Jafar TH, Stark PC, Schmid CH, et al.** Progression of chronic kidney disease: the role of blood pressure control, proteinuria, and angiotensin-converting enzyme inhibition: a patient-level meta-analysis. Ann Intern Med. 2003;139:244-52.

15. **Lewis EJ, Hunsicker LG, Bain RP, Rohde RD.** The effect of angiotensin-converting-enzyme inhibition on diabetic nephropathy. The Collaborative Study Group. N Engl J Med. 1993;329:1456-62.

16. **Elias MF, Wolf PA, D'Agostino RB, et al.** Untreated blood pressure level is inversely related to cognitive functioning. The Framingham Study. Am J Epidemiol. 1993;138:353-64.

17. **Launer LJ, Masaki K, Petrovitch H, et al.** The association between midlife blood pressure levels and late-life cognitive function. The Honolulu-Asia Aging Study. JAMA. 1995;274:1846-51.

18. **Forette F, Seux ML, Staessen JA, et al.** Systolic Hypertension in Europe Investigators. The prevention of dementia with antihypertensive treatment: new evidence from the Systolic Hypertension in Europe (Syst-Eur) study. Arch Intern Med. 2002;162:2046-52.

19. **Lithell H, Hansson L, Skoog I, et al.** The Study on Cognition and Prognosis in the Elderly (SCOPE): principal results of a randomized double-blind intervention trial. J Hypertens. 2003;21:875-86.

20. **Kannel WB, Abbott RD, Savage DD, et al.** Epidemiologic features of chronic atrial fibrillation. The Framingham study. New Engl J Med. 1982;306:1018-22.

21. **Krahn AD, Manfreda J, Tate RB, et al.** The natural history of atrial fibrillation: incidence, risk factors, and prognosis in the Manitoba Follow-Up Study. Am J Med. 1995;98:476-84.

22. **Healey JS, Connolly SJ.** Atrial fibrillation: hypertension as a causative agent, risk factor for complications, and potential therapeutic target. Am J Cardiol. 2003; 91:9G-14G.

23. **Chaturvedi N, Sjolie AK, Stephenson JM, et al.** Effect of lisinopril on progression of retinopathy in normotensive people with type 1 diabetes. The EUCLID Study Group. EURODIAB controlled trial of lisinopril in insulin-dependent diabetes mellitus. Lancet. 1998;351:28-31.

8

■ ■ ■

Hypertension and Kidney Disease

Dave C.Y. Chua, MD, MSc

George L. Bakris, MD

C hronic kidney disease is a major public health problem in the United States and is the most common identifiable cause of hypertension, present in 2%-5% of hypertensive patients (1). The Third National Health and Nutrition Examination Survey (NHANES III) estimates that 5.6 million Americans aged 17 or older have decreased renal function. The most common cause of renal insufficiency in the western world is diabetes. In more than 85% of such patients, blood pressure (BP) values are above 140/90 mm Hg.

Hypertension and macroalbuminuria are common diagnoses in more than 80% of patients starting maintenance dialysis. The management of hypertension in kidney disease is challenging and generally requires at least three different and complementary acting anti-hypertensive medications to achieve the recommended BP goal of less than 130/80 mm Hg. This concept has been captured in the Seventh Report of the Joint National Committee on Prevention, Detection, Evaluation, and Treatment of High Blood Pressure (JNC-7) guidelines. These guidelines are also consistent with recommendations by the National Kidney Foundation and the American Diabetes Association for preservation of kidney function and reduction in cardiovascular risk in people with kidney disease (2).

Definitions

Nephropathy is divided into five stages based on glomerular filtration rate (GFR) and starts at a GFR of less than 90 mL/min (Table 8-1) (3). Decreased

Table 8-1   Stages and Prevalence of Chronic Kidney Disease (Age ≥ 20)

Stage	Description	GFR (mL/min/1.73 m²)	Prevalence N (1000s)	%
1	Normal	>90	10,259	5.8
2	Mild	60-89	21,794	12.3
3	Moderate	30-59	5,910	3.3
4	Severe	15-29	363	0.2
5	Kidney failure	<15 or dialysis	300	0.15

kidney function is defined as elevated serum creatinine concentration (1.6 mg/dL or higher in men and 1.4 mg/dL or higher in women). It is important to note that people younger than age 60 years with serum creatinine of 1.5 mg/dL or higher and those older than age 60 years with a creatinine 1.3 mg/dL or higher have already lost at least 30% of their kidney function (1).

Microalbuminuria, defined as a level of urine albumin between 30 and 299 mg/g creatinine, in a spot urine is a major cardiovascular risk factor and a hallmark of diabetic renal disease (4). It is strongly associated with an increased cardiovascular risk in hypertensive people but does not usually predict nephropathy progression in nondiabetic kidney disease (4). Proteinuria defined as higher than 300 mg albumin/gram creatinine in a spot morning urine signifies renal disease and is strongly associated with an increased risk for kidney disease progression. This is especially true at levels of proteinuria higher than 1 gm per day (5).

The National Kidney Foundation's Proteinuria, Albuminuria, Risk Assessment, Detection, and Elimination (PARADE) task force reviewed the evidence relating proteinuria and microalbuminuria to renal and cardiovascular risk (6). Recent long-term clinical trials in patients who have lost more than 35% of their kidney function, with or without diabetes, demonstrate that reductions in proteinuria by 30% or more below initially measured levels are associated with marked reductions in the progression of renal disease (7). However, at present, there are no clinical outcome studies that have established proteinuria as an independent indication for therapy.

Treatment

Treatment Goals

Epidemiological data demonstrate that BP levels in the pre-hypertensive and Stage 1 range are associated with higher cardiovascular event rates (Figure 8-1). Thus, it makes sense that early treatment of stage 1 hypertension may

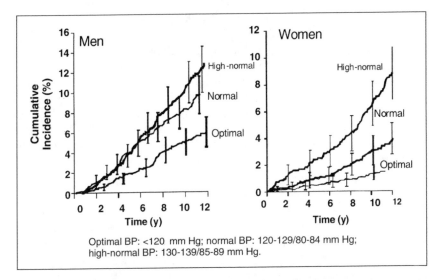

Optimal BP: <120 mm Hg; normal BP: 120-129/80-84 mm Hg;
high-normal BP: 130-139/85-89 mm Hg.

Figure 8-1   Impact of high-normal BP on CV disease risk.

be protective against development of both cardiovascular disease and progressive renal failure, although no single trial to date in this cohort has
tested this hypothesis. Post-hoc analyses of more than a dozen trials
demonstrate a lower cardiovascular event rate and a slower decline in
kidney function in the groups with systolic BP of lower than 140 mm Hg as
compared with those that are 10 mm Hg or higher (7). However, a recent
double-blind, placebo-controlled trial in more than 1000 participants with
hypertensive nephrosclerosis in African Americans did not find a significant
advantage in further slowing renal disease progression by lowering systolic
BP to lower than 130 mm Hg versus being in the range of 130-139 mm Hg
(8). Nevertheless, the national and international guidelines for goal BP for
patients with renal disease and/or diabetes as outlined by JNC-7, the
American Diabetes Association, the National Kidney Foundation, and the
Canadian Hypertension Society is lower than 130/80 mm Hg (2,9). These
recommendations are largely driven by data from patient-level meta-analyses. In one such meta-analysis, systolic BP goals of 110-129 mm Hg were
found to markedly slow progression of kidney disease in patients with proteinuria of more than 1.0 g/day (5). In this analysis, those with protein excretion of more than 2-3 g/day, lowering the diastolic pressures by less
than 80 mm Hg demonstrated optimal renal protection.

Non-Pharmacologic Strategies

Lifestyle modifications offer the potential to moderate hypertension and
should always be encouraged. These lifestyle modificiations, which are discussed in detail in Chapter 5, include dietary sodium restriction (2-4 g/day),

reduced alcohol consumption (maximum 2 oz of alcohol per day), weight reduction to avoid obesity (BMI <30), ingestion of high potassium foods such as fruits and vegetables, regular aerobic exercise (walking 30 minutes at a good pace 4 to 5 times per week), and smoking cessation (2).

Sodium retention is the major pathophysiological mechanism that contributes to hypertension development in chronic renal disease. This is particularly important in African Americans because they excrete a lower sodium load, and hypertensive blacks demonstrate greater angiographic and histological evidence of arteriolar nephrosclerosis than whites (10). In addition, excessive dietary sodium intake attenuates the protective effects of angiotensin-converting enzyme (ACE) inhibitors, angiotensin-receptor blockers (ARBs), and calcium antagonists (CAs). For these reasons, reducing dietary sodium intake is essential to the overall treatment plan of patients with hypertension associated with chronic kidney disease, including those receiving therapy with antihypertensive drugs.

Pharmacologic Strategies

The general approach of pharmacologic management to achieve goal BP is summarized in Figure 8-1. This represents an integrated approach that combines the recommendations of the National Kidney Foundation and the JNC-7 guidelines. Based on data of BP goals in the setting of an outpatient general medicine clinic, it is apparent that if an individual's BP is greater than 20/10 mm Hg above the desired BP goal, then two different antihypertensive agents should be started simultaneously to achieve the goal (i.e., either an ACE inhibitor or an ARB with a thiazide diruetic) (2). Generally, the number of antihypertensive agents needed to achieve the recommended goal BP of lower than 130/80 mm Hg is three.

ACE Inhibitors and/or ARBs
All guidelines indicate that antihypertensive agents with the ability to reduce BP and microalbuminuria and/or macroalbuminuria are preferred first-line agents to preserve renal function. A logical approach to reduce BP and macroalbuminuria in nondiabetic renal disease is to initiate therapy with an ACE inhibitor, with the dose titrated upward to the moderate-high range (20-40 mg of lisinopril or equivalent). Keep in mind that in clinical outcome trails of renal insufficiency, high doses of ACE inhibitors and ARBs were used with the greatest benefits. Thus, maximal doses of ARBs and moderate doses as noted above of ACE inhibitors should be used in renal insufficiency to obtain benefits seen in trials. This is also supported by another meta-analysis that showed a 31% reduced risk of end-stage renal disease with ACE inhibitor–based treatment over other regimens in more than 1100 people (11). Diabetics with the most advanced nephropathy generally have severe macroalbuminuria and may derive the greatest benefit from BP reduction with ACE inhibitors or ARBs (12).

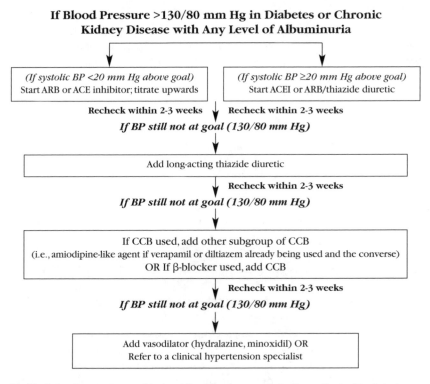

If Blood Pressure >130/80 mm Hg in Diabetes or Chronic Kidney Disease with Any Level of Albuminuria

(If systolic BP <20 mm Hg above goal)
Start ARB or ACE inhibitor; titrate upwards

(If systolic BP ≥20 mm Hg above goal)
Start ACEI or ARB/thiazide diuretic

Recheck within 2-3 weeks   Recheck within 2-3 weeks
If BP still not at goal (130/80 mm Hg)

Add long-acting thiazide diuretic

Recheck within 2-3 weeks
If BP still not at goal (130/80 mm Hg)

If CCB used, add other subgroup of CCB
(i.e., amiodipine-like agent if verapamil or diltiazem already being used and the converse)
OR If β-blocker used, add CCB

Recheck within 2-3 weeks
If BP still not at goal (130/80 mm Hg)

Add vasodilator (hydralazine, minoxidil) OR
Refer to a clinical hypertension specialist

Figure 8-2   Approach to achieving blood pressure goals in the patient with diabetes or chronic kidney disease.

Although ACE inhibitors block formation of angiotensin-II, it can still be produced by alternate means through the chymase pathways. In spite of this increase in angiotensin II, however, BP reduction is maintained through bradykinin potentiation of ACE inhibitors. ARBs serve as a substitute for ACE inhibitors if they are not tolerated. ARBs have a specific portfolio of studies demonstrating protection against declines in kidney function among those with type 2 diabetes and nephropathy, markedly reducing the time to dialysis and transplantation. In some studies the concomitant use of an ACE inhibitor with an ARB has been shown to further reduce proteinuria; however, only one, relatively short-term study in advanced nondiabetic kidney disease has supported an effect on renal outcome (13).

Diuretics

Diuretics have consistently demonstrated their ability to reduce cardiovascular mortality and are excellent additive adjuncts to ACE inhibitors and ARBs. They are recommended by JNC-7 as the drug class that should be combined with the ARBs and ACE inhibitors. In diabetic patients, these agents are a necessary part of the antihypertensive cocktail in order to achieve the desired BP control in most clinical circumstances and have been shown to reduce cardiovascular mortality. In hypertensives with at least Stage 3 nephropathy (GFR <60 mL/min), a loop diuretic is required for optimal BP-lowering effect. A thiazide diuretic such as metolazone can be added to a loop diuretic for additional volume control or to aid in the management of hyperkalemia or edema.

Calcium Channel Blockers

When used as adjunctive therapy to ACE inhibitors or ARBs, CCBs are associated with a reduced risk for progression of kidney disease based on post-hoc analyses of the Reduction of End points in NIDDM with the Angiotensin II Antagonist Losartan (RENAAL trial) in diabetic kidney disease (14). Adding CCBs to the regimen should be considered if the BP goal has not been reached after 2 to 3 weeks of therapy with the initial agents (ACE inhibitors or ARBs with or without a diuretic).

Renoprotective effects of CCBs, especially the dihydropyridine-CCBs (DHP-CCBs) subclass, used in absence of ACE inhibitors or ARBs have not been established. Only two prospective trials have assessed the impact of initiating antihypertensive treatment with a DHP-CA. In the more than 700 participants between these trials, the DHP-CA, amlodipine, did not alter progression of kidney disease when compared with an ACE inhibitor or an ARB; in one of these studies it was similar to placebo among those with diabetic nephropathy. Conversely, in a subpopulation of African Americans with hypertensive nephrosclerosis and varying levels of proteinuria (African American Study of Kidney Disease and Hypertension [AASK] study), the deterioration of renal function in the amlodipine arm was significantly faster when compared with the ACE inhibitor. Moreover, in hypertension trials that examined people without established heart or renal disease, DHP-CCBs reduce the risk of stroke and to a lesser extent myocardial infarction, which are 10-100 times more prevalent than end-stage renal disease.

Beta-Blockers

Beta-blockers have a clear role as adjunctive therapy in patients with renal disease, primarily reducing cardiovascular events and slowing, albeit to a lesser extent than ACE inhibitors and ARBs, the progression of nephropathy. In the UKPD Study of patients with Type 2 diabetes, atenolol was as effective as captopril in both arterial pressure lowering and in protection against macrovascular and microvascular disease. Newer agents in this class, e.g. carvedilol, have been shown to reduce cardiovascular mortality and microalbuminuria without adversely affecting glucose tolerance or lipid profiles in patients with hypertension or diabetes. The combination of beta-blockers and ACE inhibitors, however, does not show any additive benefits on BP reduction, especially if the baseline pulse rate is less than 84 beats per minute.

Therapeutic Applications

An ACE inhibitor or ARB should be included as initial BP-lowering therapy and up-titrated unless contraindicated by hyperkalemia (serum [K+] ≥6 mEq/L). The optimal dose of either drug needed to maximally preserve renal function is unknown, but higher doses (e.g., captopril 50 mg three times a day, enalapril 20 mg daily, 100 mg/day, losartan, 300 mg/day, irbesartan) were used in outcome trials. Due to the little further increase in BP lowering and no side effect increase seen with ARBs, frequently starting at the maximal does in people with kidney disease is warranted (15). Clinicians should all be familiar with the different dosing schedules, and the highest appropriate dose must be considered in all patients to comply with clinical trial evidence.

Whether an ACE inhibitor or an ARB should be stopped if the serum creatinine increases above baseline is unclear. A 30%-35% increase in serum creatinine (baseline <3 mg/dL) within the first 4 months of starting therapy or reducing BP toward the goal of <130/80 mm Hg with ACE inhibitor or ARB are positive prognostic signs that correlate with reduction of the progression of renal disease (2,16). (It is assumed that serum potassium is maintained <6.0 mEq/L and the rise in Cr stabilizes after this 4-month period.) However, if within the first 2 months of starting ACE inhibitors or ARBs serum Cr rises by more than 30%-35% in the absence of heart failure and continues to rise, chronic volume depletion or bilateral renal artery stenosis need to be ruled out.

Patients with renal disease, especially those on maintenance dialysis, take an average of 11 different medications daily. Combination antihypertensive medications, such as an ACE inhibitor or an ARB combined with either a diuretic or a CCB, may be useful in reducing the pill burden as well as co-payments at managed care pharmacies. If these combinations fail to achieve the BP goal, addition of other agents should be considered (Figure 8-2). Long-acting combinations are also likely to improve patient medication adherence in addition to BP control, resulting in a more consistent and cost-effective management of hypertension. Lastly, combinations of two different subclasses of CAs should be considered if BP is not controlled before minoxidil is contemplated. Three separate studies have shown that the combination of low doses of a DHPCA with a non-DHPCA provide synergistic reductions in BP (17).

■　■　■

Key Points

- The goal BP for people with chronic renal insufficiency is <130/80 mm Hg. Use of three to four different antihypertensive medications is frequently necessary and is warranted to achieve such goals.

- People less than 60 years of age with a serum creatinine of >1.5 mg/dL and those at or over age 60 with a creatinine of >1.3 mg/dL should be considered as having lost substantial amounts of kidney function.

- An ACE inhibitor or an ARB should be included as initial BP-lowering therapy and up-titrated unless contraindicated by hyperkalemia (serum [K+] >6 mEq/L).

- Agents that lower BP and albuminuria (e.g., ACE inhibitors, ARBs) are preferred to those that only lower BP in people with kidney disease.

- Diuretics are excellent additive adjuncts to ACE inhibitors and ARBs.

- CCBs, when used as adjunctive therapy to ACE inhibitors or ARBs, are associated with a reduced risk for progression of kidney disease.

- A 30% increase in serum creatinine (baseline <3 mg/dL) within the first 4 months of BP-lowering therapy with an ACE inhibitor or ARB in the absence of hyperkalemia (serum [K+] >6 mEq/L) is a postivie prognostic sign of slowed progression of renal disease. A rise of >30%, in the absence of heart failure, especially within the first 2 months of starting these agents, clearly indicates volume depletion or, if BP is significantly reduced, bilateral renal artery stenosis.

■   ■   ■

REFERENCES

1. **Coresh J, Astor BC, Greene T, et al.** Prevalence of chronic kidney disease and decreased kidney function in the adult US population. Third National Health and Nutrition Examination Survey. Am J Kidney Dis. 2003;41:1-12.

2. **Chobanian AV, Bakris GL, Black HR, et al.** The Seventh Report of the Joint National Committee on Prevention, Detection, Evaluation, and Treatment of High Blood Pressure: the JNC 7 report. JAMA. 2003;289:2560-72.

3. K/DOQI clinical practice guidelines for chronic kidney disease: evaluation, classification, and stratification. Kidney Disease Outcome Quality Initiative. Am J Kidney Dis. 2002;39:S1-246.

4. **Garg JP, Bakris GL.** Microalbuminuria: marker of vascular dysfunction, risk factor for cardiovascular disease. Vasc Med. 2002;7:35-43.

5. **Jafar TH, Stark PC, Schmid CH, et al.** Progression of chronic kidney disease: the role of blood pressure, proteinuria, and angiotensin-converting enzyme inhibition. A patient-level meta-analysis. Ann Intern Med. 2003;39:244-52.

6. **Keane WF, Eknoyan G.** Proteinuria, albuminuria, risk, assessment, detection, elimination (PARADE): a position paper of the National Kidney Foundation. Am J Kidney Dis. 1999;33:1004-10.

7. **Garg J, Bakris GL.** Treatment of hypertension in patients with renal disease. Cardiovasc Drug Ther. 2002;16:503-10.

8. **Wright JT, Jr., Bakris G, Greene T, et al.** Effect of blood pressure lowering and antihypertensive drug class on progression of hypertensive kidney disease: results from the AASK trial. JAMA. 2002;288:2421-31.

9. 2003 European Society of Hypertension-European Society of Cardiology guidelines for the management of arterial hypertension. J Hypertens. 2003;21:1011-53.

10. **Wilson DK, Sica DA, Miller SB.** Effects of potassium on blood pressure in salt-sensitive and salt-resistant black adolescents. Hypertension. 1999;34:181-6.

11. **Jafar TH, Stark PC, Schmid CH, et al.** Proteinuria as a modifiable risk factor for the progression of non-diabetic renal disease. Kidney Int. 2001;60:1131-40.

12. **Gaede P, Vedel P, Larsen N, et al.** Multifactorial intervention and cardiovascular disease in patients with type 2 diabetes. N Engl J Med. 2003;348:383-93.

13. **Nakao N, Yoshimura A, Morita H, et al.** Combination treatment of angiotensin-II receptor blocker and angiotensin-converting-enzyme inhibitor in non-diabetic renal disease (COOPERATE): a randomised controlled trial. Lancet. 2003;361:117-24.

14. **Bakris GL, Weir MR, Shanifar S, et al.** Effects of blood pressure level on progression of diabetic nephropathy: results from the RENAAL study. Arch Intern Med. 2003;163:1555-65.

15. **Weinberg MS, Kaperonis N, Bakris GL.** How high should an ACE inhibitor or angiotensin receptor blocker be dosed in patients with diabetic nephropathy? Curr Hypertens Rep. 2003;5:418-25.

16. **Bakris GL, Weir MR.** Angiotensin-converting enzyme inhibitor-associated elevations in serum creatinine: is this a cause for concern? Arch Intern Med. 2000;160:685-93.

17. **Bakris GL, Williams M, Dworkin L, et al.** Preserving renal function in adults with hypertension and diabetes: a consensus approach. National Kidney Foundation Hypertension and Diabetes Executive Committees Working Group. Am J Kidney Dis. 2000;36:646-61.

18. K/DOQI clinical practice guidelines on hypertension and antihypertensive agents in chronic kidney disease. Am J Kidney Dis. 2004;43:1-290.

19. **Vasan RS, Larson MG, Leip EP, et al.** Impact of high-normal blood pressure on the risk of cardiovascular disease. N Engl J Med. 2001;345:1291-7.

9

■ ■ ■

Future Considerations for Antihypertensive Therapy: Lessons from Outcome Trials

William J. Elliott, MD, PhD

ypertension may be the therapeutic area in medicine for which treatment recommendations are most easily supported by outcomes-based clinical trials. Trial results have been, and will continue to be, used by expert panels such as the Joint National Committee on Prevention, Detection, Evaluation, and Treatment of High Blood Pressure (JNC) to shape guidelines for clinical practice (1). Since 1967,when the results of the first Veterans' Administration Trial were published, impressive progress has been made in hypertension. Many of the changes in the attitudes and prescribing habits of American physicians were stimulated by the results of outcomes-based clinical trials. Even as late as 1958, some professors of medicine taught that "essential hypertension" was necessary because the kidney required such high pressures for proper perfusion and that lowering blood pressure (BP) was deleterious. When 27 of 70 veterans suffered terminating events (including four deaths) during placebo treatment compared with one non-debilitating stroke (and no deaths) among 73 patients treated with drugs in the first VA trial, this position was no longer tenable.

In the late 1970s, a "normal" BP was often defined as "100 + age" over 90 mm Hg or lower; many authorities feared that drug treatment of hypertension in older people could be dangerous. Since the results of the Systolic Hypertension in the Elderly Program (SHEP) and other clinical trials became known, we no longer have age-based definitions of hypertension, and antihypertensive drug treatment has become one of the most common therapies for older Americans.

Therapeutic Lifestyle Changes

Expert panels have nearly uniformly recommended non-drug therapies to lower BP. Many of these, especially in the short term, do lower BP (see Table 9-1), but no outcomes-based clinical trial data show that they are effective in reducing cardiovascular morbidity or mortality, which is the goal of treating hypertension (1).

Although non-drug approaches that lower BP have been used for primary *prevention* of hypertension, many of them are also recommended as definitive or adjunctive treatments for hypertension (1,2). Many clinical trials of the non-drug approaches have been conducted in hypertensive people, rather than in individuals with BPs lower than 140/90 mm Hg. Their results are perhaps easiest to discuss when summarized in a meta-analysis. A systematic review (18 trials, 2611 patients) of dietary advice for

---

Table 9-1   Lifestyle Modifications for Prevention and Treatment of Hypertension

Modifications That Lower Blood Pressure
- Attain and maintain normal body weight for adults (BMI, 18.5-24.9 kg/m^2)
- Reduce dietary sodium intake to no more than 100 mmol/d (approximately 6 g of sodium chloride or 2.4 g of sodium per day)
- Engage in regular aerobic physical activity, such as brisk walking (at least 30 minutes per day, most days of the week)
- Limit alcohol consumption to no more than 1 oz (30 mL) of ethanol (e.g., 24 oz [720 mL] of beer, 10 oz [300 mL] of wine, or 3 oz [90 mL] of 80-proof spirits) per day in most men, and no more than 0.5 oz (15 mL) of ethanol per day in women and lighter-weight persons
- Maintain adequate intake of dietary potassium (>90 mmol [3500 mg] per day)
- Consume a diet that is rich in fruits and vegetables and in low-fat dairy products with a reduced content of saturated and total fat (e.g., the Dietary Approaches to Stop Hypertension [DASH] diet)

Modifications That Are Routinely Recommended
- Avoid tobacco (lowers cardiovascular risk independently of any effect on blood pressure)
- Consume fish (improves lipid profile and reduces cardiovascular risk more than blood pressure–lowering effect could)
- Increase dietary fiber (improves lipid profile and reduces cancer risk, independently of any effect on blood pressure)

Modifications That Are Not Routinely Recommended
- Biofeedback
- Dietary calcium supplementation
- Dietary magnesium supplementation
- Micronutrient supplementation

Adapted from Whelton PK, He J, Appel IJ, et al. Primary prevention of hypertension: clinical and public health advisory from the National High Blood Pressure Education Program. JAMA 2002;288:1882-8; with permission.

weight loss indicates that a 3%-9% weight reduction correlated with an approximately 3 mm Hg systolic and diastolic BP reduction (3). A systematic review (58 trials, 2161 patients) of salt restriction indicated that reduction of dietary sodium chloride by 118 mmol/day lowers BP by about 3.9/1.9 mm Hg (both P <0.001) (4). The effect (both of dietary sodium and BP reduction) appears to be somewhat diminished with longer-term follow-up (5).

Perhaps the most interesting of the clinical trials comparing various therapeutic lifestyle changes for preventing hypertension was published in 1992 (6). In the 10-center Trials of Hypertension Prevention, Phase I, 2182 men and women aged 30-54 years, with diastolic BPs between 80 and 89 mm Hg were randomized to seven different non-pharmacological therapies or placebo. Despite excellent adherence to protocol and expert advice, there were no significant decreases in diastolic BP over 6 months in those randomized to stress management, calcium, magnesium, potassium, or fish oil supplements. On the other hand, weight loss (on average, 3.9 kg, P <0.01) was associated with a significant decrease in diastolic BP (approximately 2.3 mm Hg) after 18 months. This was numerically superior to the significant (P <0.05) 0.9 mm Hg reduction in diastolic BP seen with sodium restriction (on average, urinary sodium decreased by 44 mmol/day). These data, and those from several previous and later trials, indicate that the single most effective lifestyle intervention to reduce diastolic BP is weight loss.

The combination of weight loss and sodium restriction was more effective than either modality alone after 6-12 months in the subsequent Trials of Hypertension Prevention, Phase II. Weight loss and sodium restriction were also compared in hypertensive people who were removed from their previous antihypertensive drug therapy in the Trial of Non-Pharmacologic Interventions in the Elderly (TONE) study (7). Advice about weight loss and sodium restriction *combined* was more significantly effective than either alone (or neither) in maintaining BP <140/90 mm Hg or having a cardiovascular event over 30 months of follow-up. The educational programs implemented in TONE and TOHP were both quite manpower-intensive; savings from fewer drug purchases would probably be outweighed by the costs of visits for advice regarding therapeutic lifestyle changes and BP monitoring in most organized systems of medical care today.

The Treatment of Mild Hypertension Study is the only long-term treatment trial with cardiovascular events that incorporated very intensive and expert advice about lifestyle modification (8). Lifestyle modification therapy was delivered alone or with antihypertensive drug therapy for an average of 4 years in 902 slightly hypertensive young people. Although the study was underpowered for its primary outcome event (only coronary heart disease events), there was a significant difference (P = 0.03) between lifestyle modifications alone and the group receiving additional drug therapy (when pooled) in total cardiovascular events (which included stroke and other cardiovascular death). These data indicate that antihypertensive drug therapy *plus* therapeutic lifestyle changes are significantly more effective in reducing major cardiovascular events in hypertensive persons than the drug therapy alone. Expert panels recommend lifestyle modification as an initial approach for pre-hypertensive patients and as adjunctive therapy to drugs in hypertensive patients because it can be implemented without direct medical supervision and its attendant costs.

Placebo or No Treatment vs. Various Active Drug Therapies

In the early years of antihypertensive drug therapy, it was still ethical to give placebo (or no treatment) to some patients in long-term clinical trials involving cardiovascular outcomes. Although this is no longer the case, one can use the older data to compare various antihypertensive drug classes as initial therapy against placebo or no treatment (Figure 9-1). Initial treatment with a low-dose diuretic (5 trials, 15,086 patients), angiotensin-converting enzyme (ACE) inhibitor (6 trials, 23,141 patients), or calcium antagonist (6 trials, 11,508 patients) was more effective in preventing stroke, myocardial infarction (MI), and cardiovascular death than placebo or no treatment (9,10). An initial beta-blocker (6 trials, 21,076 patients) significantly prevented only stroke, but not MI or cardiovascular death (9). A

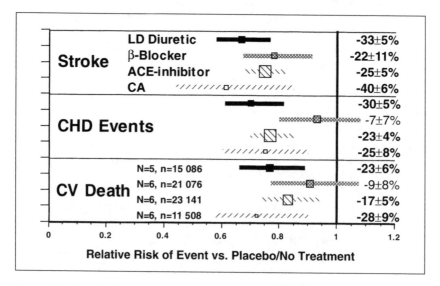

Figure 9-1 Results of a meta-analysis of various initial drug therapies against placebo or no treatment. LD = low dose; ACE = angiotensin-converting enzyme; CA = calcium antagonist; CHD = coronary heart disease; CV = cardiovascular; N = number of trials; n = number of patients.

very similar conclusion was reached in a meta-analysis of only 2 trials (4199 patients) that used beta-blockers as initial drug therapy against placebo in patients older than 60 years of age, in which only stroke was significantly prevented (11). In contrast, in the analysis of older patients, an initial low-dose diuretic (8 trials, 12,537 patients) provided significant benefit in preventing *all* types of major cardiovascular events, compared with placebo (11).

Compelling Indications

Many clinical trials have recently demonstrated major cardiovascular benefits with certain antihypertensive drug therapies when given to patients with specific medical conditions (Table 9-2). In some of these studies, the specific agents were tested against placebo, while in others another antihypertensive agent was used as an "active control." The latter is generally a stronger study design because it allows (if the results are positive) an attribution of benefit to the drug tested that extends "beyond BP lowering." Because most studies with active comparators were not successful in reducing BP to the same degree, concerns are often expressed when the group with lower BP (even by a few mm Hg) has significantly better outcomes. A recent meta-regression analysis that included all 44 trials (269,981 patients) published through March 2003 concluded that all outcome differences across drug treatments could be explained by achieved differences in systolic BP (12).

Heart Failure

A wide variety of antihypertensive drugs have been proven in clinical trials to reduce morbidity and mortality in patients with heart failure. In 1997, JNC-VI recognized ACE inhibitors and diuretics as having proven value in this setting. Since then, multiple clinical trials with low-dose beta-blockers (including carvedilol, metoprolol, and bisoprolol) have demonstrated major significant improvements in prognosis in heart failure patients treated with ACE inhibitors with or without diuretics. In addition, spironolactone (at target doses of only 25 mg twice daily) reduced all-cause mortality by 30% when added to "standard therapy," which typically included an ACE inhibitor, diuretic, and digoxin. More recently, it was found that the angiotensin II receptor blockers (ARBs), valsartan and candesartan, improve morbidity or mortality, compared with placebo, when added to "standard therapy," which included an ACE inhibitor in most patients studied. Each drug significantly improved survival (compared with placebo) in people who were unable to tolerate an ACE inhibitor, which is the setting for which valsartan received FDA approval for heart failure.

Table 9-2   Compelling Indications for Which Specific Antihypertensive Drug Therapy Reduced Morbidity and Mortality in Clinical Trials

Compelling Indication	Treatment Prevents/Delays	Recommended in 1997	Recommended in 2003
Heart failure (systolic type)	CV Events	ACE-I (CONSENSUS, SAVE, etc.)	β-Blockers (MERIT-HF, etc.); spironolactone (RALES); ARB (Val-HeFT; CHARM)
After recent myocardial infarction (MI)	Recurrent infarction or death	β-Blocker (ISIS, etc.)	
Diminished LV function after recent MI	Recurrent infarction, CHF hospitalization	ACE-I (SAVE, TRACE)	Eplerenone (EPHESUS)
Known CV disease	CV events		ACE-I (HOPE, EUROPA)
Type 1 diabetes mellitus	Deterioration in renal function	ACE-I (CCSG)	
Type 2 diabetes	CV events		ACE-I (MICRO-HOPE)
Type 2 diabetic nephropathy	Deterioration in renal function		ARBs (IDNT, RENAAL)
Type 2 diabetes	Progression of microalbuminuria		ACE-I (MICRO-HOPE); ARB (IRMA-2)
Older hypertensive persons	CV events	Diuretic (SHEP); DHP-CA (Syst-Eur)	ACE-I or DHP-CA (STOP-2); DHP-CA (Syst-China); ARB (SCOPE, second-line); ARB (LIFE)
Non-diabetic renal impairment	Deterioration in renal function		ACE-I (REIN, AIPRI, AASK); ARB + ACE-I (COOPERATE)
Prior stroke/TIA	Stroke and CV events		ACE-I (PROGRESS)
LVH (using strict criteria)	CV events (perhaps limited to stroke)		ARB (LIFE)

ACE-I = angiotensin converting-enzyme inhibitor, ARB = angiotensin receptor blocker, DHP-CA = dihydropyridine calcium antagonist.
CONSENSUS = COoperative North Scandinavian ENalapril SUrvival Study (N Engl J Med.1987;316:1429-1435); SAVE = Survival And Ventricular Enlargement study (N Engl J Med. 1992;327:669-677); CCSG = Captopril Cooperative Study Group (N Engl J Med. 1993;323:1456-1462); SHEP = Systolic Hypertension in the Elderly Program (JAMA, 1991;265:3255-3264); Syst-Eur = Systolic Hypertension in Europe trial (Lancet. 1997;360:757-764); MERIT-HF = MEtoprolol Randomized Intervention Trial in congestive Heart Failure (JAMA, 2000;283:1295-1302); RALES = Randomized Aldactone Evaluation Study (N Engl J Med. 1999;341:709-717); Val-HeFT = Valsartan Heart Failure Trial (N Engl J Med. 2001;345:1667-1675); CHARM =
(Cont'd)

Candesartan in Heart failure: Assessment of Reduction in Morbidity and mortality (Lancet, 2003;362:759-766); ISIS = International Study of Infarct Survival (Lancet, 1986;2:57-66); TRACE = TRAndolapril Cardiac Evaluation (N Engl J Med., 1995;333:1670-1676); EPHESUS = Eplerenone Post-myocardial infarction Heart Failure Efficacy and Survival Study (N Engl J Med., 2003;348:1309-1321); HOPE = Heart Outcomes Prevention Evaluation (N Engl J Med., 2000;342:145-153); EUROPA = EUropean Reduction Of cardiac events with Perindopril in stable coronary Artery disease (Lancet, 2003;362:782-788); MICRO-HOPE = MIcroalbuminuria, Cardiovascular and Renal Outcomes substudy of the Heart Outcomes Prevention Evaluation (Lancet, 2000;355:253-259); IDNT = Irbesartan Diabetic Nephropathy Trial (N Engl J Med. 2001;345:841-860); RENAAL = Reduction of Endpoints in Non-Insulin Dependent Diabetes Mellitus with the Angiotensin II Antagonist Losartan (N Engl J Med. 2001;345:861-869); IRMA-2 = Irbesartan Microalbuminuria study #2 (N Engl J Med., 2001;345:870-878); STOP-2 = Swedish Trial in Old Patients with hypertension #2 (Lancet, 1999;354:1751-1756); Syst-China = Systolic Hypertension in China trial (J Hypertens. 1998;16:1823-1829); SCOPE = Study on COgnition and Prognosis in the Elderly; LIFE = Losartan Intervention for Endpoint Reduction (Lancet, 2002;359:995-1003); REIN = Ramipril Evaluation In Nephropathy trial (Lancet, 1998;352:1252-1256); AIPRI = Angiotensin-converting-enzyme Inhibition in Progressive Renal Insufficiency (Kidney Int., 1997;Suppl. 63:S63-S67); AASK = African American Study of Kidney disease and hypertension (JAMA. 2002;288:2421-2431); COOPERATE = Combination treatment of angiotensin-II receptor blocker and angiotensin-converting enzyme inhibitor in non-diabetic renal disease (Lancet. 2003;361:117-124); PROGRESS = Perindopril pROtection aGainst REcurrent Stroke Study (Lancet, 2001;358:1033-1041).

Post-Myocardial Infarction

For patients who have had a recent MI, a beta-blocker has been recommended for more than 20 years to prevent death and recurrent infarction. An ACE inhibitor improves prognosis (even when a beta-blocker is administered) when there is evidence of heart failure at presentation or diminished left ventricular function during or after the index infarction. The Eplerenone Post-Acute Myocardial Infarction Heart Failure Efficacy and Survival Study (EPHESUS) trial randomized 6644 patients post-MI with left ventricular dysfunction to either eplerenone, a selective aldosterone blocker, or placebo, in addition to conventional therapy (including, in most patients, an ACE inhibitor, beta-blocker, and aspirin). The group randomized to eplerenone had significant benefits in mortality and either mortality or hospitalization for cardiovascular disease (13).

Known Cardiovascular Disease

An ACE inhibitor can be recommended for patients with previous cardiovascular events or interventions, based on The Heart Outcomes Prevention Evaluation (HOPE) study (14). In this important clinical trial, a full-dose ACE inhibitor (ramipril, 10 mg/d) or placebo was added to whatever drug regimen was deemed appropriate by the investigator; only ACE inhibitors or ARBs were prohibited. Approximately 52% of the 9297 enrolled subjects had a history of a prior MI, approximately 80% had known coronary heart disease, and about 11% had a prior stroke or transient ischemic attack (TIA). The study was stopped earlier than its planned 5-year follow-up because of overwhelming benefit of the ACE inhibitor: a 22% reduction in the composite cardiovascular endpoint (first MI, stroke, or cardiovascular death). BP was not carefully monitored during the study, and some individuals took ramipril at bedtime. Despite these departures from standard medical practice, the authors chose to attribute the impressive benefits seen in the trial to the randomized drug, rather than to the approximate 3/2 mm Hg reduction in BP associated with it. This interpretation has not been universally accepted.

Diabetes Mellitus

In 1997, JNC-VI recommended the prevention of end-stage renal disease (ESRD) in Type 1 diabetics as a "compelling indication" for an ACE inhibitor. This was based on the Captopril Cooperative Study Group's results that showed a reduction in the time to doubling of serum creatinine, as well as a highly significant 50% reduction in death, dialysis, or transplantation with captopril (compared with placebo).

Since then, a number of important clinical trials extend this early recommendation to ACE inhibitors (to prevent cardiovascular events) and ARBs (to prevent progression of renal disease in Type 2 diabetics). The Myocardial Infarction, Cerebrovascular, and Renal Outcomes substudy of the Heart Outcomes Prevention Evaluation (MICRO-HOPE) showed the benefits of an ACE inhibitor, ramipril (at 10 mg/d), compared with placebo. The 3577 diabetics in the HOPE study all had existing vascular disease or at least one other risk factor for cardiovascular disease. The primary outcome measure was (as in the parent HOPE study), a composite of MI, stroke, or cardiovascular death, and was reduced by 25% (P <0.001) among those given ramipril. In addition, each individual component of the primary endpoint was significantly (P <0.001) reduced by ramipril: MI (22%), stroke (33%), and cardiovascular death (37%). Those who received the ACE inhibitor also enjoyed a 24% reduction in all-cause mortality, a 17% reduction in revascularization procedures, and a 24% reduction in having proteinuria >300 mg/d. This last endpoint is particularly important in Ontario, Canada (where HOPE was designed and coordinated) because in that province physicians receive a supplemental payment for office visits for diabetics who excrete more than 300 mg/d of protein. In MICRO-HOPE, however, there were only 18 individuals who developed end-stage-renal disease: 10 in the placebo group and 8 among those given ramipril. Because of the small numbers, however, this 30% reduction (according to the time-to-event analysis) was not statistically significant. These data suggest that diabetics had major benefits associated with the use of ramipril vs. placebo. DIABHYCAR, a very similarly designed trial in Type 2 diabetics that used only 1.25 mg/d of ramipril, showed no benefit over placebo.

The benefits of angiotensin II receptor blockers in Type 2 diabetics have been demonstrated in three important clinical trials reported in 2001. Although lower BP has been commonly associated with reduced rates of ESRD, diabetes has been the most commonly cited diagnosis leading to

ESRD in the United States since the early 1980s. Two groups of investigators therefore decided in early 1995 to test the efficacy of an ARB in preventing the progression of diabetic nephropathy. Both studies used a identical primary endpoint: doubling of serum creatinine, ESRD, or all-cause mortality. The Irbesartan Diabetic Nephropathy Trial (IDNT) enrolled 1715 people with a 15-year history of diabetes, BP of 159/87 mm Hg, a serum creatinine of about 1.7 mg/dL, and 24-hour urinary protein excretion of 2.9 gm/d. They were randomized to irbesartan (average dose 269 mg/d), amlodipine (average dose 9.1 mg/d), or placebo. Other drugs (3-4 on average but not including ACE inhibitors, calcium antagonists, or ARBs, by design) were added, as needed, to lower BP (to 142/78 mm Hg on average). The study was ended prematurely because of emerging evidence of major benefit with inhibitors of the renin-angiotensin system in diabetics. Irbesartan was associated with a 20% reduction in the primary endpoint (vs. placebo, $P = 0.02$) and a 23% reduction compared to amlodipine ($P = 0.006$). Because the enrolled patients already had diabetic nephropathy at enrollment, they were at much higher risk for ESRD than for cardiovascular events; as a result, this may have precluded finding a significant difference across randomized groups in cardiovascular events.

Very similar results were found in the Reduction of Endpoints in Non-Insulin-Dependent Diabetes Mellitus with the Angiotensin II Antagonist Losartan (RENAAL) study. In this trial, 1513 Type 2 diabetics with an average BP of 152/82 mm Hg and a serum creatinine of 1.9 mg/dL were randomized to losartan or placebo and then given 2.5 (on average) other antihypertensive drugs (excluding ACE inhibitors or ARBs) to achieve an average BP of 141/74 mm Hg. For losartan compared to control, there was a 16% reduction in the primary endpoint (with the *exact same* P-value as was seen in IDNT study), a 25% reduction in doubling serum creatinine, and, perhaps most impressively, a 23% reduction in institution of dialysis or kidney transplantation. Both irbesartan and losartan have now been approved by the FDA for delaying the progression of Type 2 diabetic nephropathy.

The cardiovascular benefits of an ARB (compared with a beta-blocker) were demonstrated in the diabetic substudy of the Losartan Intervention for Endpoint (LIFE) reduction trial. LIFE enrolled hypertensive patients with very strictly defined left ventricular hypertrophy (LVH), including 1195 diabetics (15). After approximately 5 years of follow-up, the diabetics assigned to losartan had a significant 27% (unadjusted) or 24% (adjusted for baseline differences in LVH and Framingham risk score) risk of the composite endpoint of MI, stroke, or cardiovascular death. Unlike the overall LIFE results, the diabetics assigned to losartan had significantly fewer cardiovascular events, demonstrating that ARBs *do* have significant cardiovascular benefits in Type 2 diabetics.

Like ACE inhibitors, ARBs also reduce the risk of microalbuminuria progression (typically defined as 30-299 mg/d of protein in a 24-hour urine collection) to frank proteinuria (≥300 mg/d) in diabetics. The Irbesartan MicroAlbuminuria-2 (IRMA-2) trial randomized 590 Type 2 European diabetics with microalbuminuria to placebo, medium-dose (150 mg/d), or high-dose (300 mg/d) irbesartan. After 2 years, there were significantly fewer people with the primary endpoint (≥288 mg/d of proteinuria *and* an increase by more than 15% over baseline) in the high-dose ARB over placebo; the medium-dose ARB showed an intermediate response that was not significantly better than placebo.

The combination of an ACE inhibitor and an ARB has also been carefully studied in diabetics. Data from the Candesartan and Lisinopril Microalbuminuria (CALM) trial using half-maximal doses of each showed a superior BP reduction than either drug alone and a significant reduction in proteinuria compared with the ARB alone (but not compared with the ACE inhibitor alone, perhaps due to a lack of statistical power). More data about the combination of full-dose ARB and full-dose ACE inhibitor in diabetics are expected soon.

Older Patients

In JNC-VI, diuretics were recommended as initial therapy for older patients with isolated systolic hypertension, primarily based on the Systolic Hypertension in the Elderly Program (SHEP). Long-acting dihydropyridine calcium antagonists were considered an alternative, based on the Systolic Hypertension in Europe (Syst-EUR) trial.

Since 1997, additional recommendations can be made based on several other trials. The Syst-China study used a very similar study design to Syst-EUR, but (for cultural reasons) used sequential allocation rather than randomization to assign drug therapy. The results of Syst-China were very similar to Syst-EUR: the antihypertensive regimen beginning with nitrendipine (a long-acting dihydropyridine calcium antagonist) had a 38% reduction in stroke (compared with 42% seen in Syst-EUR). The second Swedish Trial of Older Persons with Hypertension randomized 6614 hypertensives over age 70 to either a diuretic or a beta-blocker, one of two dihydropyridine calcium antagonists, or one of two ACE inhibitors. After 6 years of follow-up, the major adverse cardiovascular event rates were nearly identical across the three randomized groups. These data support the previous recommendations for dihydropyridine calcium antagonists as useful antihypertensive therapy in older people with hypertension, although the ALLHAT data (and others) indicate that similar results occur with initial diuretic therapy, which has a lower acquisition cost.

Three recent trials have explored the role of ARBs for older hypertensive persons, with mixed results. The subset of 1326 participants in the LIFE study (average age, 70 years) with isolated systolic hypertension had fewer cardiovascular events if randomized to losartan compared with atenolol, despite a nearly-identical reduction in BP. The Study on Cognition and Prognosis in the Elderly (SCOPE) gave either candesartan or placebo to 4937 European patients aged 70-89 years whose BP was still elevated despite 12.5 mg/d of hydrochlorothiazide. Neither ARBs nor ACE inhibitors were allowed as concomitant therapy, but any other antihypertensive drug was acceptable during the 3.5 years of follow-up. BP was significantly lower in the group assigned to the ARB (decrease of 22/11 vs. 18/9 mm Hg), and major adverse cardiovascular events were also slightly (but not significantly) lower (238 vs. 266, $P = 0.19$). Nonfatal stroke was significantly reduced in the ARB group, but this benefit was balanced by more nonfatal MI.

The Valsartan Long-Term Use Evaluation randomized 15,256 patients with an average age of 67 years to valsartan or amlodipine, followed by a diuretic. Larger BP reductions were noted, especially in the first few months of follow-up, in the group given amlodipine. After 4.2 years, there were no significant differences between groups in cardiac morbidity/mortality, although MI was significantly lower in the group given amlodipine. Trends favoring amlodipine for these endpoints, as well as stroke and all-cause mortality, were seen early during follow-up and generally diminished over time, lending support to the hypothesis that early blood pressure control plays an important role in event prevention.

We are likely to have much more information about drug treatment of isolated systolic hypertension soon, as data about patients with this important public health problem who were included in recently completed clinical trials are published. As compared with placebo or no treatment, however, a meta-analysis from the INDANA group showed that drug treatment of isolated systolic hypertension in eight clinical trials significantly reduced stroke by 30%, coronary heart disease events by 23%, all cardiovascular events by 26%, and all-cause mortality by 13%.

Non-Diabetic Renal Impairment

Several clinical trials have recently demonstrated the benefit of ACE inhibitors in preventing or delaying the onset of ESRD in non-diabetic renal disease. Two lesser-known European studies compared placebo with either ramipril or benazepril. In the Ramipril Efficacy in Nephropathy (REIN) trial, 97 patients with non-diabetic renal disease were randomized to either ramipril or placebo, then given other antihypertensive drugs (excluding ACE inhibitors or ARBs). After 6 years of follow-up, there was a 46% reduction in ESRD or death ($P = 0.02$) in the group randomized to ramipril. In the larger Angiotensin-Converting-Enzyme Inhibition in Progressive Renal Insufficiency (AIPRI) study, 583 patients with mostly non-diabetic renal disease (n=562) were given either placebo or benazepril, along with whatever non-ACE inhibitor or non-ARB antihypertensive drugs were required. The original report showed a significant reduction of doubling of serum creatinine,

ESRD, or death (31 vs. 57, P <0.001) at 3 years of follow-up; longer observation (average 6 years) showed persistence of prevention of ESRD or death, despite mandatory discontinuation of placebo. These and nine similar trials of ACE inhibitors have been combined in meta-analysis, which allowed identification of non-use of ACE inhibitor, proteinuria >1 g/d, and systolic BP lower than 110 or higher than 130 mm Hg as major risk factors for progression of non-diabetic kidney disease.

African Americans have a much higher risk of ESRD than whites, even apart from diabetes. As a result, the African American Study of Kidney Disease (AASK) and hypertension was organized to determine which initial antihypertensive drug therapy was most effective in reducing the time-dependent decrease in glomerular filtration rate (GFR). One thousand ninety-four patients with hypertensive nephrosclerosis were randomized (in a 2:1:2 ratio) to an ACE inhibitor (ramipril), calcium antagonist (amlodipine) or beta-blocker (metoprolol succinate), and followed for 3-5 years. The amlodipine arm was discontinued early because it was significantly inferior to the ACE inhibitor, both in chronic decrease in GFR and renal events (41% reduction in ESRD or death, P = 0.007). After an average of 4 years of follow-up, the ACE inhibitor was superior to the beta-blocker (16). These data extend the conclusions of the European studies and show that, despite a higher risk of cough and angioedema with ACE inhibitors in African Americans, these drugs are very helpful in preventing the decline in renal function in non-diabetic renal disease.

ARBs alone have not been extensively studied in non-diabetic renal disease, but recently the combination of full-dose ACE inhibitor (defined as the threshold dose beyond which proteinuria decreased no further; 3 mg/d of trandolapril) and full-dose ARB was compared with either therapy alone in Japanese patients. Although there was no better BP lowering, the combination showed a significant reduction in proteinuria and about half the incidence of doubling of serum creatinine or ESRD (P = 0.017) than either full-dose monotherapy.

Post-Stroke or Post-Transient Ischemic Attack

For many years, there was reluctance to use antihypertensive drugs for patients who had recently suffered a stroke or TIA. This policy arose from early observations of acute BP lowering in post-stroke patients, in whom the neurological deficit sometimes worsened. Although controversy still exists, both the HOPE and Perindopril Protection Against Recurrent Stroke Study (PROGRESS) have demonstrated benefits of an ACE inhibitor in this population. In the HOPE study, the 1013 individuals with a previous stroke or TIA enjoyed a (non-significant) 13% reduction in recurrent stroke if randomized to ramipril. More specific was the PROGRESS study, in which 6105 patients from 10 countries with a history of stroke or TIA within the previous 5 years were randomized to either perindopril (with or without indapamide, a diuretic) or placebo (with or without another placebo). The intent was to have all patients taking both antihypertensive drugs, but investigators were allowed to withhold the diuretic if there was concern about hypotension or other adverse effects of the combination. Those randomized to the ACE inhibitor had a 9/4 mm Hg lower BP than the placebo group, enjoyed a significant 28% reduction in recurrent stroke, and had a 26% reduction in major adverse cardiovascular events. The recurrent stroke benefit was significant and independent of baseline BP. However, a post-hoc analysis showed a non-significant 7% benefit on recurrent stroke among those who received only the ACE inhibitor (i.e., without the diuretic).

This observation has been variously interpreted but may have resulted from an "indication bias" that occurred because low-risk people preferentially did not receive the combination of the ACE inhibitor and the diuretic. The data from both HOPE and PROGRESS support a policy to lower BP in the long-term (using an ACE inhibitor) for patients with a prior stroke or TIA. More recently, the Acute Candesartan Cilexetil Evaluation in Stroke Survivors (ACCESS) study gave candesartan to 342 patients either 1 or 7 days post-stroke; those receiving candesartan only a day after the neurological event had significantly better 1-year event-free survival.

Left Ventricular Hypertrophy

Although LVH has long been recognized as a major cardiovascular risk factor (probably because it results most commonly from a prolonged period of undertreated or uncontrolled hypertension), only recently have clinical trials enrolled patients with this condition, to see if regression of LVH and prevention of cardiovascular disease events are inter-related. The LIFE study enrolled 9193 hypertensive patients who had a very strict electrocardiographic definition of LVH (the Cornell voltage-duration criteria, which involves not only high voltage, but also a prolonged QRS duration) (15). Participants were randomized to 50 mg of either losartan or atenolol, and then hydrochlorothiazide was added in about 85% of participants, and thereafter any other antihypertensive drug except ACE inhibitors, ARBs, or beta-blockers. Over nearly 5 years of follow-up, the losartan group had a lower BP (by 1.3/0.4 mm Hg). The primary outcome was a composite of first MI, stroke, or cardiovascular death; the differences across randomized treatments were "adjusted" in a Cox model for baseline differences in the degree of LVH and Framingham risk score. The results were interpreted as being the first to show that "it matters how BP is lowered," as there was a 13% (adjusted) reduction in the composite primary event in the losartan group. This was largely due to a 25% decrease in stroke; the cardiovascular death rates were slightly (but not significantly) lower (by 11%) with the losartan group. Surprisingly, despite the presence of LVH (evidence of cardiac pathology) in each participant, the incidence of the cardiac component of the composite endpoint (heart attack) was lower (by 7%) in the atenolol group. Adverse events, new diabetes, and improvement in LVH were all significantly lower in the losartan group.

Comparisons of Various Initial Therapies in a Wide Range of Hypertensive Patients

Most of the recent trials done in a wide range of hypertensive patients comparing initial drug therapies involved diuretics/beta-blockers, calcium antagonists, or ACE inhibitors. The only data about an initial alpha-blocker come from ALLHAT (17). The doxazosin arm of ALLHAT was discontinued prematurely; the alpha-blocker arm had a significant 10% increase in combined coronary heart disease events and a 2.04-fold increase in heart failure. Alpha-blockers have therefore been removed from the list of recommended initial antihypertensive drugs since January 2000, when this result was announced.

The many comparative studies of initial antihypertensive agents have been collected in several meta-analyses, in order to overcome the possibility of Type II statistical error inherent in many clinical trials. Since the publication of the final reports of ALLHAT, ANBP-2, AASK, CONVINCE, INVEST, and other recent trials, there is a great deal more information available about the relative merits of various antihypertensive drugs (16,18-21). Some of these data have been combined in a "network meta-analysis," which concluded that a low-dose diuretic was more effective for most cardiovascular events than other initial drug therapies (22). The WHO/ISH Blood Pressure Trialists' Collaboration analyzed patient-level data from 7 sets of 29 randomized trials (162,341 patients) and concluded that all commonly-used antihypertensive agents reduce major cardiovascular events, with larger reductions in BP leading to larger reductions in risk (24).

Estimates of the relative efficacy of antihypertensive drug classes in reducing cardiovascular events are imprecise because of the lack of complete information in the published reports (e.g., major cardiovascular events in ALLHAT, IDNT or AASK), and because the meta-analytic method combines the numbers of events, and ignores their timing (i.e., no time-to-event analyses are possible). A summary of an original meta-analytic comparison of an initial calcium antagonist vs. an initial diuretic or beta-blocker (12 trials, 92,566 patients, now including INVEST) is shown in Figure 9-2. The incidence of heart failure (not yet reported from ELSA) was 29% more common with the initial calcium antagonist, which was associated with a barely significant reduction in the risk of stroke. A summary of a meta-analysis of an initial ACE inhibitor vs. an initial diuretic or beta-blocker (7 trials, 48,287 patients) is shown in Figure 9-3. As in ALLHAT, the

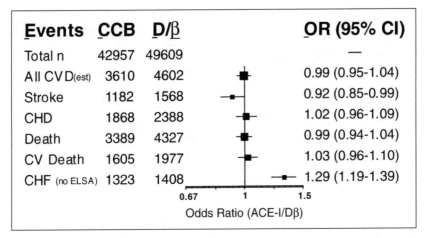

Events	CCB	D/β		OR (95% CI)
Total n	42957	49609		—
All CVD(est)	3610	4602		0.99 (0.95-1.04)
Stroke	1182	1568		0.92 (0.85-0.99)
CHD	1868	2388		1.02 (0.96-1.09)
Death	3389	4327		0.99 (0.94-1.04)
CV Death	1605	1977		1.03 (0.96-1.10)
CHF (no ELSA)	1323	1408		1.29 (1.19-1.39)

Odds Ratio (ACE-I/Dβ)

Figure 9-2 Results of a meta-analysis of 12 trials (92,566 patients) comparing an initial calcium antagonist with an initial diuretic or beta-blocker. The sizes of the boxes (representing point estimates) are proportional to the number of events for each endpoint. Although not yet reported for ELSA, the major significant ($P < 0.001$) difference was in heart failure, which was 29% more common with the initial calcium antagonist. The 8% reduction in risk of stroke was barely statistically significant ($P = 0.03$). *The number of major CV events for ALLHAT and INVEST was estimated from data given in the papers. CA = calcium antagonist; D/β = diuretic or beta-blocker; CV = cardiovascular; CHD = coronary heart disease; CHF = congestive heart failure.

diuretic/beta-blocker group had a significantly lower risk of both stroke and heart failure, the most common reason Medicare beneficiaries enter the hospital in the United States. The data from both figures support the recommendations of JNC-7, the ALLHAT Collaborative Research Group, and Psaty et al. that a diuretic should be the preferred choice for initial antihypertensive therapy (1,18,22).

Comparisons of Different Blood Pressure Targets

A systematic review (5 trials, 22,982 patients) indicated that the risk of stroke, coronary heart disease, and major cardiovascular events was reduced by 23%, 5%, and 15%, respectively, in the group receiving more intensive treatment; these benefits were more obvious in high-risk patients (e.g., diabetics) (23). One clinical trial (1094 patients) found no benefit in hypertensive African Americans randomized to a BP target of about <125/75 mm Hg, as opposed to approximately <140/90 mm Hg (16). These results support the original recommendation in JNC-VI and subsequently other guidelines for a lower target BP in diabetics but suggest that a much lower BP for patients with renal disease and major proteinuria is not very effective in reducing renal endpoints (1).

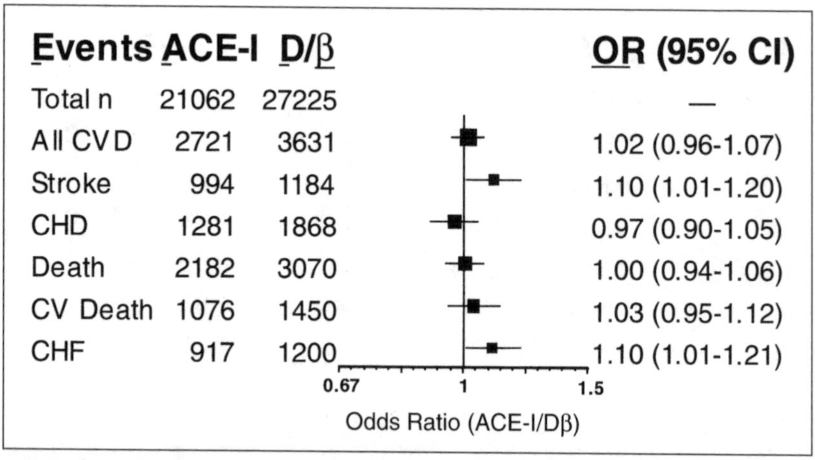

Events	ACE-I	D/β		OR (95% CI)
Total n	21062	27225		—
All CVD	2721	3631		1.02 (0.96-1.07)
Stroke	994	1184		1.10 (1.01-1.20)
CHD	1281	1868		0.97 (0.90-1.05)
Death	2182	3070		1.00 (0.94-1.06)
CV Death	1076	1450		1.03 (0.95-1.12)
CHF	917	1200		1.10 (1.01-1.21)

Odds Ratio (ACE-I/Dβ)

Figure 9-3   Results of a meta-analysis of 7 trials (48, 287patients) comparing an initial ACE inhibitor and an initial diuretic or beta-blocker. The sizes of the boxes (representing point estimates) are proportional to the number of events for each endpoint. The number of patients included in the meta-analysis for stroke, CHD events, and CHF is reduced because data from AASK and HYVET regarding these parameters have not yet been publicly revealed. Both strokes and heart failure events were just barely significantly (P = 0.04) more common with the ACE inhibitor, compared with the diuretic or beta-blocker; this may change when the missing data from AASK and HYVET are included. *Numbers of major CV Events for ALLHAT were estimated from data given in the paper. ACE-I = angiotensin converting-enzyme inhibitor, D/β = diuretic or beta-blocker; CV = cardiovascular; CHD = coronary heart disease; CHF = congestive heart failure.

Ongoing and Future Outcome-Based Clinical Trials

A wide variety of outcome-based clinical trials have already begun or are in the late planning stages (Table 9-3). Although these may help us to understand the relative benefits of some of the new therapies, especially ARBs, they are unlikely to change the recommendation to use a diuretic as the initial drug therapy in most patients.

■ ■ ■

Key Points

- The two major therapeutic lifestyle changes that reduce blood pressure in clinical trials are weight loss and sodium restriction. These are recommended as definitive or adjunctive modalities to reduce BP but have never been shown in clinical trials to reduce cardiovascular morbidity and mortality.

Table 9-3   Ongoing and Future Outcomes-Based Clinical Trials

Acronym (Name)	Test Agent	Comparator	Patients	Comments
ASCOT (Anglo-Scandinavian Cardiac Outcomes Trial)	Amlodipine ± Perindopril	Atenolol ± Bendrofluazide	19,342 residents of Scandinavia or the U.K.	5-year follow-up planned; primary outcome: fatal or non-fatal MI
ACCOMPLISH (Avoiding Cardiovascular events through COMbination therapy in Patients Living with Systolic Hypertension)	Benazepril + Amlodipine	Benazepril + HCTZ	~12,600 patients with SBP > 160 mm Hg, and D < 115 mm Hg	Event-driven, but 5-year follow-up expected; two primary outcomes: CVD morbidity, CVD mortality
HYVET (Hypertension in the Very Elderly Trial)	Indapamide ± Perindopril	Placebo	~2,100 patients > 80 years old	5-year follow-up planned; primary outcome: fatal or non-fatal stroke
ON-TARGET (ONgoing Telmisartan Alone and in Combination with Ramipril Global Endpoint Trial)	Telmisartan + Ramipril	Telmisartan or Ramipril	~23,400 patients with established vascular disease, but no heart failure	5.5-year follow-up planned; primary outcome: CVD death, MI, stroke, hospitalization for CHF
TRANSCEND (Telmisartan RANdomized assessment Study in ACE-I iNtolerant patients with cardiovascular Disease)	Telmisartan	Placebo	Patients with established vascular disease, intolerant of ACE-inhibitors, but no heart failure	5.5-year follow-up planned; primary outcome: CVD death, MI, stroke, hospitalization for CHF
TROPHY (TRial of Prevention of HYpertension)	Candesartan	Placebo	803 Persons with high-normal blood pressure	4-year follow-up planned; primary outcome: incident hypertension

- Many antihypertensive drugs have been proven to prevent morbidity and/or mortality in clinical trials in other conditions. Specific drug therapy can therefore be easily recommended if a person with hypertension has one of these conditions.

- An initial diuretic, ACE inhibitor, or calcium antagonist significantly prevents a wide variety of major cardiovascular endpoints compared with placebo or no treatment.

- In updated meta-analyses of large comparative clinical trials, an initial diuretic or beta-blocker significantly prevented heart failure better than an ACE inhibitor, a calcium antagonist, or an alpha-blocker.

- On the basis of clinical trial data, a lower-than-usual goal blood pressure can be recommended for diabetic patients with hypertension; this goal is currently <130/80 mm Hg.

- Future trials of antihypertensive drugs are likely to extend the number of compelling indications for these drugs and may revise the currently recommended order of administration (diuretic, followed by beta-blocker or ACE inhibitor, or possibly a calcium antagonist or angiotensin II receptor blocker).

■   ■   ■

REFERENCES

1. **Chobanian AV, Bakris GL, Black HR, et al.** The Seventh Report of the Joint National Committee on Prevention, Detection, Evaluation, and Treatment of High Blood Pressure: The JNC-7 Report. JAMA. 2003;289:2560-72.

2. **Whelton PK, He J, Appel LJ, et al.** Primary prevention of hypertension: clinical and public health advisory from the National High Blood Pressure Education Program. JAMA. 2002;288:1882-8.

3. **Mulrow CD, Chiquette E, Angel L.** Dieting to reduce body weight for controlling hypertension in adults. Cochrane Review. Oxford, UK: Update Software, Volume 2, 2004.

4. **Graudal NA, Galloe AM, Garred P.** Effects of sodium restriction on blood pressure, renin, aldosterone, catecholamines, cholesterols, and triglycerides: A meta-analysis. JAMA. 1998;279:1383-91.

5. **Hooper L, Bartlett C, Davey Smith G, Ebrahim S.** Systematic review of long-term effects of advice to reduce dietary salt in adults. BMJ. 2002;325:628.

6. **Trials of Hypertension Prevention Collaborative Research Group.** The effects of nonpharmacologic interventions on blood pressure of persons with high normal levels: Results of the Trials of Hypertension Prevention, Phase I. JAMA. 1992;267:1213-20.

7. **Whelton PK, Appel LJ, Espeland MA, et al.** Sodium reduction and weight loss in the treatment of hypertension in older persons: a randomized controlled trial of nonpharmacologic interventions in the elderly (TONE). JAMA. 1998;279:839-46.

8. **Neaton JD, Grimm RH Jr, Prineas RJ, et al.** Treatment of Mild Hypertension Study: final results. Treatment of Mild Hypertension Study Research Group. JAMA. 1993;270:713-24.

9. **Psaty BM, Smith NL, Siscovick DS, et al.** Health outcomes associated with anti-hypertensive therapies used as first-line agents: a systematic review and meta-analysis. JAMA. 1997;277:739-45.

10. **Elliott WJ.** Cardiovascular events during long-term antihypertensive drug treatment: meta-analysis of four major drug classes vs. placebo or no treatment [Abstract]. Am J Hypertension. 2003;16:113A.

11. **Messerli FH, Grossman E, Goldboourt U.** Are beta-blockers efficacious as first-line therapy for hypertension in the elderly: a systematic review. JAMA. 1998;279:1903-7.

12. **Staessen JA, Wang J-G, Thijs L.** Cardiovascular protection and blood pressure reduction: a quantitative overview updated until 1 March 2003. J Hypertension. 2003;21:1055-76.

13. **Pitt B, Remme W, Zannad F, et al.** Eplerenone Post-Acute Myocardial Infarction Heart Failure Efficacy and Survival Study Investigators. Eplerenone, a selective aldosterone blocker, in patients with left ventricular dysfunction after myocardial infarction. N Engl J Med. 2003;348:1309-21.

14. **The Heart Outcomes Prevention Evaluation Study Investigators.** Effects of an angiotensin-converting enzyme inhibitor, ramipril, on death from cardiovascular causes, myocardial infarction, and stroke in high-risk patients. N Engl J Med. 2000;342:145-53.

15. **Dahlöf B, Devereux RB, Kjeldsen SE, et al.** The LIFE study group. Cardiovascular morbidity and mortality in the Losartan Intervention for Endpoint reduction in hypertension study (LIFE): a randomised trial against atenolol. Lancet. 2002; 359:995-1003.

16. **Wright JT Jr., Bakris GL, Greene T, et al.** Effect of blood pressure lowering and antihypertensive drug class on progression of hypertensive kidney disease: results from the AASK Trial. JAMA. 2002;288:2421-31.

17. **The ALLHAT Collaborative Research Group.** Major cardiovascular events in hypertensive patients randomized to doxazosin vs. chlorthalidone: the Antihypertensive and Lipid-Lowering Treatment to Prevent Heart Attack Trial (ALLHAT). JAMA. 2000;283:1967-75.

18. **The ALLHAT Officers and Coordinators for the ALLHAT Collaborative Research Group.** Major outcomes in high-risk hypertensive patients randomized to angiotensin-converting enzyme inhibitor or calcium channel blocker vs. diuretic. The Antihypertensive and Lipid Lowering Treatment to Prevent Heart Attack Trial (ALLHAT). JAMA. 2002;288:2981-97.

19. **Wing LMH, Reid CM, Ryan P, et al.** Second Australian National Blood Pressure Study Group. A comparison of outcomes with angiotensin-converting-enzyme inhibitors and diuretics for hypertension in the elderly. N Engl J Med. 2003;348:583-92.

20. **Black HR, Elliott WJ, Grandits G, et al** for the Controlled Onset Verapamil Investigation of Cardiovascular Endpoints Investigators. Principal results of the Controlled Onset Verapamil Investigation of Cardiovascular Endpoints (CONVINCE) trial. JAMA. 2003;289:2073-82.

21. **Pepine CJ, Handberg EM, Cooper-DeHoff RM, et al.** A calcium antagonist vs. a non-calcium antagonist hypertension treatment strategy for patients with coronary artery disease: the International Verapamil-Trandolapril Study (INVEST). A randomized controlled trial. The INVEST Investigators. JAMA, 2003;290:2805-16.

22. **Psaty BM, Lumley T, Furberg CD, et al.** Health outcomes associated with various antihypertensive therapies used as first-line agents: a network meta-analysis. JAMA. 2003;289:2534-44.

23. Effects of different blood-pressure-lowering regimens on major cardiovascular events: results of prospectively-designed overviews of randomised trials. Blood Pressure Lowering Treatment Trialists' Collaboration. Lancet, 2003;362:1527-35.

10

■　■　■

Secondary Hypertension

Domenic A. Sica, MD

Secondary hypertension must always be identified because treatment will be based on the specific underlying disorder. Secondary hypertension differs most notably from essential hypertension in that an etiology can be identified, its onset is often sudden, it may be more severe, a family history is frequently absent, and it may occur in patients of all ages. Specific symptoms may help guide the diagnosis for many causes of secondary hypertension.

Secondary hypertension can emerge in connection with such diverse endocrine disorders as primary hyperaldosteronism or pheochromocytoma. In addition, secondary hypertension can develop in association with co-morbid conditions such as sleep apnea, panic disorders, and/or depression. It can also develop in conjunction with a variety of medications, including nonsteroidal anti-inflammatory drugs (NSAIDs), oral contraceptives (OCPs), and sympathomimetic amines, and with excessive alcohol intake. Finally, secondary hypertension can be linked to renal abnormalities such as renal artery stenosis and/or progressive renal parenchymal disease (Table 10-1).

Diagnosis

Initial Approach

Secondary hypertension is often found on top of pre-existing hypertension. Secondary hypertension diagnoses come from a long list of possibilities unique to the mindset and experience of an individual physician. For example, a pulmonary specialist might think nothing about routinely diagnosing sleep apnea as a contributor to a hypertensive state, whereas an internist may consider it rare and therefore low on his list of possibilities. Panic-related hypertension may be not uncommonly seen by a psychiatrist, but it may be exceedingly difficult to identify in a busy internist's office practice.

Table 10-1   Clues to Secondary Forms of Hypertension

Renal parenchymal disease	Increased urine creatinine, active urine sediment, small kidneys on renal ultrasound
Renal vascular disease	Abrupt onset of hypertension at age <30 or >55 years, systolic/diastolic abdominal bruit, unilateral small kidney, unexplained rise in serum creatinine, or a sudden increase in serum creatinine with an ACE inhibitor
Pheochromocytoma	Headache, palpitations, and sweating, BP volatility, orthostatic hypotension, increased urinary catecholamines, often confused with panic disorder
Cushing's syndrome	Truncal obesity, moon facies, buffalo hump, hyperglycemia, plasma cortisol >5 ug/dL at 8 a.m. after 1 mg of dexamethasone at 11 p.m. the evening before
Primary aldosteronism	Hypokalemia, spontaneous or provoked, muscle cramps, weakness, aldosterone-to-renin ratio >30
Sleep apnea	Obesity, male gender, prominent snoring, daytime somnolence
Panic disorders	Mimics pheochromocytoma, profound constitutional symptoms

The inventory of secondary causes of hypertension tends to be arbitrary, but secondary causes should be investigated, particulary in the case of the resistent hypertensive. A resistant hypertensive is generally defined as having inadequate blood pressure (BP) control despite three maximally titrated medications. Resistant hypertensives should undergo 24-hour ambulatory blood pressure monitoring (ABPM) during the course of their work-up. One in four patients with apparent resistant hypertension will be found to have controlled BP.

Secondary hypertension may account for a significant proportion of resistant hypertensives (10%-30%), particularly those referred into tertiary care centers. Resistance to treatment in a compliant patient may provide the prompt to undertaking a systematic evaluation for secondary causes of hypertension. Table 10-1 outlines clinical clues to the presence of the more common secondary causes of hypertension.

Evaluation

A thorough, well-structured evaluation should be made. Table 10-2 provides a helpful approach by addressing initial common causes of resistant hypertension for which secondary causes of hypertension should be suspected. A careful history should always address prior and current medication use, including herbal medicines, recreational drugs, and over-the-counter (OTC) substances such as sympathomimetic amines and NSAIDs. Whenever a patient is questioned, the clinician should be remember that many patients are not forthcoming about OTC medication use. In younger women, OCP

Table 10-2   Sequential Steps in Approaching Refractory Hypertension*

Step 1. Is the prescribed regimen adequate, appropriate, and well-tolerated?

Step 2. Are drug-drug interactions possible?

Step 3. Consider pseudoresistance including the possibility of volume expansion and/or renin-angiotensin-aldosterone axis activation

Step 4. Is the patient adherent with the prescribed regimen?

Step 5. Empiric modification of the regimen to include individualized and targeted therapy

Step 6. Consider secondary forms of hypertension with targeted hemodynamic and neurohumoral assessment

---

* It is presumed for Step 1 that the prescribed regimen is inadequate for the patient to be labeled a refractory hypertensive. Step 4 is not sequential, per se, but is determinable at any juncture. Step 6 is directed by available history, physical exam, and routine laboratory.

use should be considered. Identifying a temporal cause-and-effect relationship between a newly initiated medication and a rise in blood pressure (BP) can lessen the need for an extensive search for more occult secondary causes.

Pseudoresistance

Before embarking on a work-up for secondary hypertension, the clinician should establish that in fact, the medication regimen used has not produced pseudoresistance and/or that the prescribed regimen is being taken. Pseudoresistance is the activation of counterregulatory responses, such as tachycardia, volume expansion, and/or renin-angiotensin-aldosterone/sympathetic nervous system, sufficient to blunt the BP-lowering effect of an antihypertensive. If pseudoresistance to an antihypertensive regimen emerges, it most commonly relates to unrecognized volume overload. Volume overload sufficient to increase BP can occur with several antihypertensive classes, including centrally-acting agents, beta-blockers, and/or direct vasodilators, such as hydralazine or minoxidil.

Most clinicians recognize the relationship between volume status and BP. However, what is poorly appreciated is how slight an increase in volume is actually needed to significantly increase BP. Volume-related pseudoresistance is often present regardless of the absence of peripheral edema. Moreover, this phenomenon can progress despite simultaneous diuretic therapy, particularly if there is a mismatch between dietary sodium intake and the natriuretic response to the administered diuretic. In the instance of pseudoresistance, the empirical reduction of extracellular volume (either by increasing the dose of an existing diuretic regimen or by converting to a more potent diuretic) can effect a significant BP reduction.

Another form of pseudoresistance takes place when the renin-angiotensin-aldosterone system (RAAS) is activated. This occurs with diuretic and/or non-specific vasodilator therapy and can be established with a random plasma renin activity and plasma aldosterone determination. Sampling for these neurohumoral parameters can be obtained in an upright position and should be obtained 24 hours after the last medication dose. In most cases plasma renin activity values in excess of 2.0 ng mL/hr represent excess activity in this system and the likelihood that drugs which curtail activity in this system (such as ACE inhibitors or angiotensin receptor blockers [ARBs]) will further reduce BP. Aldosterone values in excess of 10 ng/dL usually represent a surplus of this neurohormone and provide an opportunity to specifically target aldosterone therapeutically. Contrary to popular belief, ACE inhibitors and ARBs do not reduce aldosterone values over the long-term; thus, if a reduction in aldosterone effect is desired an aldosterone receptor antagonist, such as spironolactone or eplerenone, may be necessary.

Medication Noncompliance

It cannot be overstated how important it is to establish medication compliance before a diagnostic work-up for a secondary cause of hypertension. When a careful history raises concern about compliance with a prescribed medication regimen, one can seek physical exam clues to provide evidence of medication use. Such clues are most apparent when moderate or near-maximal medication doses are in use. The lack of reflex tachycardia in a minoxidil-treated patient and/or the absence of bradycardia in a beta-blocker–treated patient can be suggestive of poor medication compliance. The same can be said for the minoxidil-treated patient without evidence of hair growth, the calcium-channel blocker (CCB)-treated patient lacking peripheral edema, or the clonidine-treated patient missing dry mouth and/or sedation.

Endocrine Disorders

Pheochromocytoma

A pheochromocytoma is a tumor of neuroectodermal origin that produces excess quantitites of catecholamines and up to 35 other physiologically active peptides. This surfeit of catecholamines causes hypertension with a constellation of signs and symptoms that can mimic those characteristic of several other medical and/or surgical disorders. Early recognition, accurate localization and appropriate management of benign pheochromocytoma nearly always result in complete cure. In as many as 40% of patients with this diagnosis, it is discovered as an incidental finding at surgery, on CT scanning, or at autopsy. If unrecognized, these tumors cause lethal disease that can lead to significant cardiovascular morbidity and mortality and particularly to sudden death during surgical and obstetric procedures.

Frequency
Pheochromocytoma is a rare form of secondary hypertension, accounting for 0.1%-0.9% of all cases of hypertension. However, its true incidence may be higher because a considerable number of pheochromocytomas are only discovered at autopsy. The highest incidence of pheochromocytoma occurs during the 4th and 5th decades of age; however, it can occur at any age. Pheochromocytomas occur in only 1%-2% of patients with neurofibromatosis, but 5%-25% of patients with pheochromocytoma have neurofibromatosis. Patients with neurofibromatosis, therefore, even with no symptoms, should be screened for pheochromocytoma.

Clinical Features
The clinical symptoms of the disease are fairly capricious depending on the predominant secretory pattern (norepinephrine or epinephrine), as well as the parallel secretion of other neurohormones. Symptoms do not correlate with the size of the tumor per se. The classic triad of symptoms that typifies pheochromocytoma is that of hypertension, headache, and excessive/generalized sweating. Other symptoms include weight loss and hyperglycemia. Different BP patterns can exist with pheochromocytoma: 1) stable, sustained hypertensive state; 2) sustained hypertensive state with intermittent hypertensive crises; (3) normotensive state with brief, sudden, and conspicuous BP elevations. The hypertensive crisis with this disease ranges from an asymptomatic state to dizziness, flushing, visual disturbances, nausea, vomiting, or an epileptic aura. Hypertensive crises are truly episodic and unpredictable but can be triggered by mechanical compression of the tumor on physical exam, exercise, postural change, micturition, and/or eating. Orthostatic hypotension is seen in more than 50% of patients with pheochromocytoma.

Differential Diagnosis
A wide spectrum of diseases can duplicate the clinical picture of pheochromocytoma, thereby complicating its diagnosis. Some of the more important mimes in this regard include paroxysmal episodes of vasodilating headaches, autonomic dysfunction, anxiety and/or panic disorders, acute hypoglycemia, and/or the intake of sympathomimetic agents.

Diagnosis
Diagnostic priority is given to patients with signs and symptoms compatible with the disease. The assay of 24-hour urinary excretion of catecholamines and their metabolites is considered the best methodological approach for screening patients in whom this disease is suspected. It is highly sensitive and specific; however urine collections are fraught with numerous difficulties. First, advances in measurement technology for determination of urinary catecholamines have overcome problems associated with earlier less sensitive methods prone to false-positive results due to interfering substances

such as alpha-methyldopa. However, several compounds should be withheld prior to sampling including tricyclic antidepressants, labetalol, levodopa, sotalol, decongestants, clonidine, and benzodiazepines. Second, the concept of periodic hormone excess is key to the appropriate evalution of patients with possible catecholamine-secreting tumors since false-negative results may be obtained if patients are assessed at times when the catecholamine-secreting tumor is hormonally inactive. For patients with episodic hypertension, the collection should start with the onset of a spell. When collected in this manner, patients with pheochromocytoma generally have urinary catecholamine or metanephrine values two- to three-fold above normal.

Alternatively, concentrations of plasma norepinephrine and epinephrine (values of 2000 pg/mL or more are considered pathognomonic) can be measured after the patient has been situated in a quiet environment and has been recumbent for at least 30 minutes. The import of values between 1000 and 2000 pg/mL can be made clear with a clonidine suppression test. This test is based on the principle that increases in catecholamines are customarily mediated through sympathetic nervous system activation. In the case of pheochromocytoma, the excess in catecholamines sidesteps the normal storage and release mechanisms; thus, clonidine would not be expected to suppress catecholamine release.

For hypertensive patients with elevated BP readings (>160/100) in whom sudden rises in BP are ill-advised, pretreatment with a calcium channel blocker may be necessary prior to this test. Abdominal CT or MRI (preferred imaging mode) is then performed as a means to tumor localization in patients with clinical and biochemical features compatible with the disease. The 123I-MIBG scintigraphic approach, which is both sensitive and specific, should be reserved for suspicion of malignant pheochromocytoma; otherwise, distant metastases are the only clues differentiating a malignant from a benign tumor.

Treatment

Surgical treatment is the only effective therapeutic approach for pheochromocytoma, be it benign or malignant. Pre-operative management includes careful attention to volume replacement (many of these patients are subclinically volume contracted) together with combined alpha and beta-blockade. After the tumor is removed, the catecholamine secretion generally reverts to normal within 1 week.

Primary Aldosteronism

Primary aldosteronism can occur at all ages, although in most reported series patients fall in the 30-50 yr age range. Its occurrence is higher than historically thought, and it is a common cause of resistant hypertension in black and white subjects. Aldosterone-producing adenomas are more common in women, whereas idiopathic hyperaldosteronism occurs more frequently in men. Symptoms are usually related to hypokalemia and/or the complications of hypertension. Primary aldosteronism should be considered in any patient with spontaneous hypokalemia, moderately severe hypokalemia induced by conventional doses of diuretics, or refractory hypertension.

Frequency

Considerable dispute exists as to the true prevalence of primary aldosteronism with proposed values as high as 10%-12%. Much of the dispute on the prevalence rate of this disorder centers on the dependability of the screening methods (aldosterone-renin ratios) employed for diagnosis. Although the true frequency of this abnormality is unlikely to be as high as 12%, it is most certainly greater than the <1.0% values reported in the 1970s.

Clinical Features

Patients with primary aldosteronism often present with little more than mild hypokalemic alkalosis and hypertension; however, if hypokalemia is severe enough weakness, cramps, polyuria, and polydipsia may be reported. Although belief held that aldosterone-producing adenomas caused token end-organ damage, recent evidence has shown this to be incorrect. Patients with this disorder have increased rates of left ventricular hypertrophy and heart failure with and without preserved systolic function. The susceptibility of the heart to damage in primary hyperaldosteronism may be related to the recently recognized profibrotic actions of aldosterone.

Differential Diagnosis

Several rare syndromes produce endocrine hypertension that mimic primary hyperaldosteronism. They are characterized by hypokalemia and hypertension with associated suppression of both renin and aldosterone. These include the syndrome of apparent mineralocorticoid excess, Liddle's syndrome, and licorice ingestion. Cushing's syndrome may also present with hypokalemia and hypertension.

Diagnosis

Diagnosis of primary aldosteronism until relatively recently was considered only in the presence of hypertension and hypokalemia. It is now obvious that this approach will miss many surgically correctable cases of primary aldosteronism in that hypokalemia may only occur in one third of all cases (Table 10-3). The diagnosis can be readily established in the patient with a serum potassium value <3.0 mEq/L, inappropriate kaliuresis (>30-35 mmol of potassium excretion), a reduced plasma renin activity (PRA) (<1.0 ng (mL/hr), and elevated plasma or urinary aldosterone values. Unfortunately, many cases of primary aldosteronism do not provide such clear diagnostic direction. In these equivocal cases, measurement of urinary aldosterone excretion during salt loading (>250 mmol excretion of sodium) can aid in

Table 10-3   Diagnostic Considerations for Primary Aldosteronism

Test	Comment
Plasma K⁺ levels	• In the hypertensive patient, 2 to 3 plasma K^+ levels should be checked taking care to avoid artifactual effects from poor sampling and/or harvesting technique. • Primary aldosteronism is more likely when hypokalemia exists but may only occur in ⅓ of all cases.
24-hr K⁺ excretion	• >30 mmol/24 hrs in the presence of hypokalemia indicates K^+ wasting in the presence of systemic hypokalemia.
Plasma aldosterone/ renin ratio	• Can be measured randomly but is best assessed in the morning (when aldosterone is naturally highest) and in the absence of antihypertensives (particularly spironolactone). • A ratio >30 is highly suggestive of primary aldosteronism.
Fludrocortisone test	• Fludrocortisone increases ECF volume; plasma aldosterone levels will remain elevated in primary aldosteronism.
Computed tomography	• Adrenal scanning to determine the presence of unilateral or bilateral disease.
Adrenal vein sampling	• Useful if imaging is negative or equivocal and surgery is contemplated.

confirming the diagnosis. An excretion rate of greater than 14 µg/24 hrs following salt-loading sets apart 95% of patients with primary aldosteronism from those with essential hypertension.

In contrast, isolated plasma aldosterone values are helpful to a limited extent in identifying this disease (60% of patients with primary aldosteronism have plasma aldosterone values that fall within the range for essential hypertension) in that they are influenced by a diurnal rhythm (highest in the morning), the presence of hypokalemia (low potassium suppresses production), and concurrent medications (ACE inhibitors and beta-blockers tend to reduce values). Finally, PRA is increasingly used as a way to index the appropriateness of a plasma aldosterone value (plasma aldosterone: PRA ratio). This ratio typically falls below 30 and when greater than 30 assumes particular diagnostic significance. Although this test is widely viewed as the screening test of choice for primary aldosteronism, there are three drawbacks to the test: 1) the inherent variability of PRA and plasma aldosterone values, even in the presence of a tumor; 2) PRA values remain suppressed or stimulated for some time after medication discontinuation, which complicates interpretation of this computation; and 3) extremely low PRA values can drive the ratio above 30 with a small change in the absolute PRA value (e.g., with a plasma aldosterone of 15 ng/dL and a PRA value of 0.5 ng (mL/hr the ratio is 30; however, a plasma aldosterone value of 15 ng/dL and a PRA value of 0.3 ng (mL/hr results in a ratio of 45).

Treatment

The different types of primary aldosteronism need to be distinguished because management varies. Unilateral adrenal adenomas are best treated surgically, by an open or a laparoscopic procedure. In the majority of operated cases the hypertension is alleviated or substantially improved. Medical therapy is indicated in patients with bilateral adrenal hyperplasia or adenomas and patients with adenomas who are poor operative risks. Medical therapy with spironolactone is usually effective in reversing the biochemical abnormalities of primary aldosteronism, but additional antihypertensive medication may be required for BP control. In particular, sustained salt-and-water depletion with aggressive diuretic therapy noticeably boosts the BP-reducing effect of spironolactone. Contrary to belief, calcium-channel blockers do not suppress aldosterone production; therefore, they fall short in correcting the primary metabolic abnormalities of this disease. The dosage of spironolactone may be limited by symptoms of gynecomastia and impotence. Eplerenone is a newer aldosterone-receptor antagonist with fewer endocrine side effects than spironolactone.

Cushing's Syndrome

Naturally occurring Cushing's syndrome can be divided into ACTH-dependent and ACTH-independent causes. In ACTH-dependent diseases, the surplus of cortisol arises from adrenal stimulation by ACTH. The source of ACTH is usually an ACTH-secreting pituitary adenoma, also known as Cushing's disease. Twenty percent of ACTH-dependent Cushing's disease cases are a result of ectopic ACTH production by a nonpituitary tumor, most commonly caused by a small cell carcinoma of the lung or carcinoid tumor of the bronchus or thymus. Most ACTH-independent cases of Cushing's disease are caused by adrenal adenoma or carcinoma. The hypertension of Cushing's syndrome can be explained by the oversupply of cortisol.

Frequency

Cushing's syndrome is a rare cause of hypertension in that it affects less than 0.1% of the population or 5 to 25 per million/per year; however, hypertension is common in Cushing's syndrome, affecting some 80% of subjects.

Clinical Features

The clinical features in Cushing's disease relate to excessive cortisol production and in some patients an excess of adrenal androgens. The typical clinical presentation of Cushing's syndrome is that of truncal obesity, including a buffalo hump, hypertension, plethoric moon facies, proximal muscle weakness/fatigue, hirsutism, emotional disturbances, and skin abnormalities (acne, purple skin striae, easy bruising). Carbohydrate intolerance or diabetes, amenorrhea, loss of libido, osteoporosis, and/or spontaneous bone fractures may also be encountered. Few patients have all of these features, but most have some blending of these signs and symptoms. Patients with ectopic ACTH excess may not exhibit the classic manifestations of cortisol excess, instead they may present with skin hyperpigmentation (2° to overproduction of melanocyte-stimulating hormone), severe hypertension, and obvious hypokalemic alkalosis.

Differential Diagnosis
The most common cause of Cushing's syndrome is iatrogenic administration of exogenous steroids. Oftentimes the obese hypertensive patient with the dysmetabolic syndrome and a Cushingoid physical appearance can be mistaken for true Cushing's syndrome. Chronic alcohol excess can lead to a Cushingoid appearance in addition to altering cortisol metabolism.

Diagnosis
The diagnosis of Cushing's syndrome can prove difficult. Although it is burdensome to perform, the determination of 24-hour urinary free cortisol is the best available test for documenting endogenous hypercortisolism. This test has 100% sensitivity and 98% specificity and a level >100 µg/24 hr is highly discriminant for Cushing's syndrome. False-positive results may, however, be obtained in non-Cushing's hypercortisolemic states such as stress, chronic strenuous exercise, polycystic ovary syndrome, psychiatric states such as depression, and malnutrition. The dexamethasone suppression test may also be used for screening. For this test, a single dose of dexamethasone (1 mg) is given at midnight, and plasma cortisol is measured next morning at 6:00 a.m. In normal subjects cortisol values will be suppressed to <5.0 µg/dL. This test is equally sensitive to the urinary free cortisol, but slightly less specific. If dexamethasone suppression testing is used for screening, urinary free cortisol is measured as a confirmatory test.

Treatment
The prognosis of untreated Cushing's syndrome is poor, with a 50% 5-year survival. The preferred approach in Cushing's syndrome is selective excision of the pituitary adenoma by transsphenoidal surgery or adrenalectomy in the case of adrenal adenomas or carcinoma. Medical management of hypercortisolism is reserved for extensive and inoperable disease. Hypertension generally remits with corrective surgery unless exposure to cortisol has been sufficiently prolonged to establish a structural basis for more permanent hypertension. Antihypertensive drug therapy in Cushingoid patients should be attentive to the risk of exacerbating hypokalemia with diuretic therapy and/or worsening depression with beta-blockers. Potassium-sparing diuretics (amiloride or spironolactone) alone or in combination sometimes control BP, reduce edema, and correct hypokalemia.

Sleep Disorders, Panic Disorders, and Depression

Sleep Disorders

Much work has focused on the link between sleep apnea and hypertension, and the evidence that suggests a underlying association between these two conditions is persuasive. Sleep apnea is common, readily diagnosed, and usually treatable. Sleep apnea syndromes comprise two related disorders, obstructive sleep apnea (OSA) and central sleep apnea (CSA). Obstructive sleep apnea (OSA) occurs in 2% of women and 4% of men. Over 50% of individuals with OSA have hypertension. Obesity is so widespread in OSA that the index of suspicion for OSA should be high in any hypertensive patient with a BMI in excess of 27 kg/m^2. Therein, OSA occurs because of repetitive episodes of upper airway occlusion during inspiration. In this regard, sleep onset is followed by a drop off in neural drive to those muscles stiffening and preserving patency of the upper airway rendering the airway more collapsible.

These individuals should be questioned thoroughly for symptoms of OSA, including snoring, witnessed apnea, irregular breathing during sleep, restless sleeping, chronic morning fatigue, frequent traffic accidents, and declines in cognitive function. Often it is the sleep partner who provides the most dependable history, especially on the subject of snoring, because the affected individual often is oblivious to the problem. If the diagnosis is suspected clinically and the patient in question has resistant hypertension, a formal sleep study may give added direction to the hypertension therapy.

Previous debate has largely focused on the interplay between OSA, obesity, and hypertension. It now appears that the potential causal association between OSA and hypertension involves both the obesity-hypertension link and an independent role of OSA in chronic BP elevation. Independent of obesity there is a dose-response association between sleep-disordered breathing at baseline and the development of new hypertension 4 years later. The odds-ratio with an apnea-hypopnea index of more than 15 events per hour at baseline is 2.89 for the occurrence of hypertension. Episodes of apnea with repeated oxygen desaturation in OSA have been shown to provoke sympathetic nervous system activation that directly elevates BP at night (non-dipping BP pattern) with lasting effects into the daytime hours. There is also a direct relationship between the severity of sleep apnea and the level of BP. Moreover, it is recently appreciated that marked daytime and nighttime fluctuations in BP accompany moderate-to-severe breathing disorders.

While obesity is known to contribute in large part to OSA, patients with OSA may independently be at risk for further weight gain; conversely, treatment of OSA can reduce body and visceral fat buildup. In this regard, patients with newly diagnosed OSA commonly have a recent history of excessive weight gain prior to diagnosis. The mechanisms of this weight gain are multifactorial and consist of a more sedentary lifestyle because of daytime somnolence as well as resistance to the appetite suppressant and metabolic effects of leptin. Poorer sleep quality with fragmentation and shorter sleep periods may play a reinforcing role in the fatigue and daytime somnolence.

Even modest weight loss (approximately 10 kg) improves sleep apnea, and successful gastric bypass may lead to complete correction of sleep apnea. Sustained and effective treatment of OSA with continuous positive airway pressure (CPAP) has been reported to lower nighttime and daytime BP in hypertensives with OSA and may also improve cardiac ischemia and heart failure symptoms. By attenuating apneas, acute CPAP therapy prevents BP surges and nocturnal sympathetic activation.

CPAP is usually delivered by a tightly fitted nasal mask. Pressures of 10 to 15 mm Hg are typically required to obliterate snoring, apneas, hypopneas, and oxygen desaturation. Compliance is the major problem with the use of CPAP. Typically there is irritation of the nasal mucosa, leading to excessive dryness and rhinitis. Improvements in the quality of sleep in OSA patients can occur as a result of a variety of positioning measures during sleep, particularly sleeping on one's side. The role of oral prostheses and surgical approaches remains to be more fully defined. Typically, these devices advance the mandible and thrust the tongue forward.

Oftentimes, CPAP does not completely correct the hypertensive state so antihypertensive therapy remains a consideration. To this end, some types of sleep apnea improve with effective treatment of hypertension. No specific class of antihypertensive drugs has yet been demonstrated to be superior for BP lowering in OSA patients. Medications that cause sedation or increase daytime somnolence should be avoided.

Panic Disorders

A BP (and pulse rate) obtained during a panic attack will typically be elevated, sometimes highly. Panic disorders in hypertensive patients not uncommonly appear as sudden discrete episodes of flushing, trembling, choking, paresthesias, sweating, and dizziness. The attacks are recurrent, may awaken the person from sleep, and are associated with anticipatory anxiety regarding another attack. Acute panic also can evoke chest pain with some patients describing severe, crushing precordial chest pain that resembles angina pectoris. Electrocardiographic changes can indicate myocardial ischemia in these patients. Hyperventilation is an important additional feature of panic disorder and can independently increase BP.

These patients frequently go to emergency rooms. In an unstructured environment, such as an emergency room, concern regarding secondary hypertension arises, prompting additional and unnecessary testing. In fact, studies investigating patients for pheochromocytoma have shown that as many as two thirds of these patients met criteria for either current or lifetime panic disorder. Panic disorder patients also tend to receive overly aggressive antihypertensive therapy. The latter will sometimes excessively reduce BP in the time period between panic attacks and present an added stimulus for repetitive panic attacks. While a diagnosis of panic disorder may precede that of hypertension, it is far more common for panic disorder to occur following the diagnosis of hypertension in that hypertension may cause panic symptoms through a "labeling" effect on the domain of psychological well-being.

Intolerance to multiple antihypertensive drugs, particularly non-drug-specific intolerance, is strongly associated with panic disorder, anxiety, and depression. Panic disorders respond to selective serotonin reuptake inhibitors (SSRIs), tricyclic antidepressants, and, for immediate symptomatic relief, alprazolam. Cognitive-behavioral psychotherapy has been found to be effective, particularly in panic patients who may not want to take medication. In addition, patients should be weaned from a repetitive and impending doom pattern of home BP monitoring. In some instances abandoning home BP monitoring is an important component of treatment.

Depression

After controlling for age and gender, almost 9% of adults with hypertension had major depression in 1999. Depression predicts a future occurrence of hypertension in normotensive subjects and increased mortality in older adults with moderate hypertension independent of other known cardiovascular risk factors. Depression can make BP resistant to therapy if coupled with a high anxiety component, weight gain, and/or sleep abnormalities. Alternatively, BP may be lowered and need for medication decreased if depression is accompanied by significant weight loss. Finally, depression has been associated with medication noncompliance. In ordinary practice newly prescribed antihypertensive medications are often quickly stopped with adverse effects often being held accountable. It is not uncommon in the patient with multiple non-specific antihypertensive medication intolerances to have various psychiatric morbidities as the basis.

Several valid and reliable screening instruments are available for use in a primary care setting to aid in the diagnosis of depression. Resistant hypertension is not included in these screening instruments. It is, however, quite reasonable to view this as one of the various symptoms characterizing depressive disorders, particularly if BP control lapses in parallel with the onset of depression. In primary care settings pharmacotherapy is the principle treatment for depression. Newer agents such as the SSRIs are more patient friendly than were older agents such as the tricyclic antidepressants. However, several medications commonly used in psychiatry and neurology are an important iatrogenic source of weight gain; thus, the weight gain potential of various antidepressants, such as mirtazapine, should be considered in the hypertensive individual with depression.

Medications

Many prescription drugs and certain over-the-counter (OTC) agents as well as a number of herbal supplements may provoke transient or sustained forms of hypertension. Drug-induced hypertension should be suspected in the following scenarios: 1) a significant and sudden increase in BP in a hypertensive subject well-controlled beforehand; 2) existence of comorbidities, such as degenerative joint disease, calling for anti-inflammatory therapy; and 3) severe episodic hypertension of an atypical nature in an otherwise young healthy patient with a clinical picture compatible with cocaine use.

The list of drugs capable of increasing BP is lengthy although very few of the compounds that find their way onto such lists cause significant chronic changes in BP with any frequency. Those compounds with a reasonable likelihood of increasing BP are listed in Table 10-4. The mechanism(s) by which medications can increase BP, although well-defined in theory, may prove more difficult to discern in the individual patient. Causal mechanisms for drug-related hypertension include salt and water retention with extracellular fluid volume expansion, increased adrenergic activity, and/or alterations in the production, release, or effectiveness of vasodilator hormones.

A thorough medication history when the status of a patient's BP has changed can occasionally identify a medication as the source. In so doing, unnecessary and sometimes expensive testing can be avoided. Having identified a possible medication contributor to resistant hypertension then requires discontinuation of the candidate substance and careful subsequent observation to make certain that BP values return to prior levels.

Two medications (or substances) warrant additional comment: NSAIDs and alcohol because of the frequency with which each contributes to either the development or worsening of existing hypertension.

Alcohol

The hemodynamic effects of alcohol have been described at least since the middle of the 19th century. The relationship between alcohol and BP for the most part depends on the amount of alcohol imbibed rather than the type of beverage. The BP pattern with alcohol is temporally distinct: 1) there may be a direct pressor effect from alcohol in regular daily drinkers; 2) in episodic (weekend) drinkers BP may increase in conjunction with the alcohol withdrawal syndrome; 3) unrelenting heavy drinking may be accompanied by enduring chronic pressor effects even after subjects have become abstinent; and 4) alcohol intake has been associated with resistance to antihypertensive medications either because of noncompliance or true interference with medication performance. With this last pattern BP control may fluctuate between excellent and poor, sometimes prompting an unnecessary work-up seeking a more unusual secondary form of hypertension.

Table 10-4   Substances Commonly Associated with the Onset of Hypertension

Medication	Mechanism	Comment	Treatment
Estrogens	Volume expansion, renin-angiotensin axis activation	More common with high-estrogen oral contraceptives (OCs); uncommon with post-menopausal replacement; may persist after discontinuation of OCs	Discontinuation of OCs; diuretic, ACE inhibitor or ARB, or CCB
NSAIDs and COX-2 inhibitors	Volume expansion, decrease in vasodilator prostaglandins	Hypertensive response more common in salt-sensitive individuals; attenuation of diuretic action; calcium-channel blocker efficacy not blunted by these compounds	Discontinuing medication or further separating medication dosing times particularly for diuretics
Sibutramine	Increase in α-adrenergic activity	↑ in BP can be counter-balanced by weight loss if it occurs in response to treatment	Combined α-β-blockade, dosage reduction
Erythropoietin	Increase in blood volume	More common when hematocrit is allowed to rise suddenly	Any drug class; reduce or hold dose of erythropoietin if BP is too high
Cocaine	Increase in α-adrenergic activity	Often associated with marked ↑ in BP; chronic ↑ in BP is uncommon	Combined α-β-blocker therapy preferred
Sympatho-mimetic agents	Increase in α-adrenergic activity	BP ↑ is greater with concomitant β-blocker therapy	Discontinuation; combined α-β-blocker or CCB preferred
Alcohol	Increased SNS activity	Dose-dependent; if the pattern of intake leads to weight gain further rises in BP may occur	Discontinuation; centrally-acting agents such as clonidine of particular utility

The effects of alcohol on BP do not appear to relate to structural changes but rather seem to correlate with neural and hormonal changes with SNS stimulation playing a major role. Any new-onset hypertensive or one with a significant worsening of existing hypertension should be questioned carefully about alcohol intake. On occasion, independent confirmation of stated intake (by family members) may be required if the index of suspicion for a greater than reported intake is high enough on the part of the physician. A number of medications can be used in the treatment of alcohol-related hypertension although abstinence (or significant moderation) remains the action of choice. Of the drug classes with a strong physiologic rationale for use centrally-acting alpha-agonists such as clonidine (particularly in its transdermal form) can prove quite useful.

Nonsteroidal Anti-Inflammatory Drugs

NSAIDs represent one of the most common medication classes associated with hypertension. NSAIDS reduce the effectiveness of most antihypertensive medications. Among the NSAIDs, older agents like indomethacin have been the most extensively studied. BP responses vary within the class of the NSAIDs; however, increases in pressure are often accompanied by peripheral edema and weight gain but not invariably so. This supports a salt-retention mechanism of hypertension associated with the loss of natriuretic prostaglandins such as PGE2. Reduction in the well-described vasodilatory effects of some prostaglandins is another proposed mechanism. COX-2 inhibitors also may encourage an increase in BP; thus, current data suggest that certain NSAIDs and COX-2 inhibitors may have destabilizing effects on BP control.

The BP increase with either NSAIDs or COX-2 inhibitors ranges from a modest clinically indeterminable change to significant enough increases to prompt an investigative work-up for secondary causes. A cause and effect relationship between an NSAID, a COX-2 inhibitor, and hypertension often becomes a diagnosis of exclusion. In so establishing a linkage, the logical progression is to discontinue the offending medication. If BP returns to baseline levels, the presumption of causality proves correct; however, it may take several days to weeks for BP values to return completely to their baseline pre-NSAID values, which confuses the assignment of causality. If therapy with NSAIDs is unavoidable, several steps can be empirically taken to minimize their effect on BP, including using the lowest dose possible, controlling dietary sodium intake, and employing calcium-channel blockers as part of the therapeutic regimen. Calcium-channel blockers are less likely to have their antihypertensive effect attenuated by co-administered NSAIDs. In addition, if diuretics are part of the therapeutic regimen, spacing the diuretic and NSAID administration several hours apart may prove helpful in lessening the negative interaction of these two drug classes.

Associated Condition: Renal Artery Stenosis

Incidence

Strictly speaking, the prevalence of renovascular hypertension (RVH) is unknown. Its reported incidence (1%-32%) relates to the population surveyed with resistant hypertensives culled from the general hypertensive population exhibiting the highest rate. Renovascular disease clusters at the extremes of age, at least as relates to the age of onset of hypertension. If the initial diagnosis of hypertension in an adult (particularly in a non-obese female with no family history of hypertension) is made prior to the age of 30, it is often as the result of fibromuscular dysplasia, whereas new-onset hypertension in a patient older than 55 should raise concern about the possibility of atherosclerotic RAS, particularly if the patient is a heavy smoker. RVH is less common in African Americans than in whites; however, in those African-Americans with a clinical picture suggestive of RAS the incidence may approach 20%.

Diagnostic Clues

Accelerated or resistant hypertension has also been linked with a high prevalence of RAS and often provides the impetus for RAS diagnostic evaluation. Finally, frequent heart failure episodes marked by sudden BP swings, and "flash" pulmonary edema (unrelated to active ischemic heart disease) can be an indication of underlying RAS.

Physical Examination

In general, the physical examination is of limited diagnostic help for detection of RAS. Evidence of coronary, cerebral, or peripheral arterial disease increases the likelihood of RAS because of the generalized nature of atherosclerosis. A systolic abdominal bruit is a common but nonspecific finding; alternatively, finding an epigastric machinery type systolic/diastolic bruit is more suggestive of RAS. A bruit with a diastolic component implies significant enough arterial narrowing to also have disrupted diastolic flow.

Renal Function and Electrolyte Abnormalities

Unprovoked and/or steadily progressive azotemia (with a normal urine sediment) offers a clue to the presence of hemodynamically significant RAS. There are also numerous reports suggesting that patients who develop acute renal failure while receiving diuretics and/or ACE inhibitors have bilateral RAS or RAS in a solitary kidney. Finally, spontaneous hypokalemia and unexplained proteinuria can be seen with RAS when the renin-angiotensin axis is highly activated.

Imaging Studies

The ideal imaging procedure should: 1) single out the main renal arteries and accessory or polar vessels, 2) confirm the hemodynamic significance of the lesion, 3) pinpoint the site of stenosis or disease, and 4) recognize related pathology (i.e., aneurysmal disease and/or renal masses) that may have some bearing on the treatment of RAS. An intravascular intravenous pyelography (IVP) would be an example of a less than ideal imaging procedure. An IVP is seldom used as a screen for RAS because of its low sensitivity and specificity (approximately 75%), the risk of contrast nephropathy, and its relatively high radiation dose. Moreover, in the presence of bilateral RAS many of the lateralizing findings characteristic of RAS may be absent, particularly if there is little difference in function between the two kidneys. In patients with indications of renovascular disease, captopril-enhanced radionuclide renal scan, duplex Doppler flow studies, and magnetic resonance angiography offer a full complement of noninvasive and sensitive screening tests.

Captopril-Enhanced Radionuclide Renal Scan
Radionuclide imaging techniques are a noninvasive and safe way of evaluating renal blood flow and excretory function. However, the renal flow scan has unacceptably high false-positive and false-negative rates. When an ACE inhibitor such as captopril (25 to 50 mg 1 hour before scanning) is added to isotope renography, the sensitivity and specificity of the test improves noticeably, especially for patients with unilateral RAS. In most instances of unilateral RAS, the GFR of the stenotic kidney falls by approximately 30% after captopril administration. Less often, the contralateral normal kidney shows an increase in GFR, urine flow, and salt excretion despite a reduction in systemic BP. These expected physiologic changes identified by renal scintigraphy within the stenotic and contralateral kidneys are the source of the asymmetry of renal function after ACE inhibition.

Patients with unilateral disease and normal renal function are best suited for a captopril renogram. The presence of significant azotemia or bilateral RAS may reduce the accuracy of captopril renography (patients with serum creatinine values >2.5 mg/dL are often excluded). Whereas the captopril renogram was once considered the noninvasive diagnostic test of choice for patients with RAS, it is now relegated to a second tier position for screening modalities with the emergence of duplex ultrasound and MRA.

Elevated PRA values are found in less than 80% of patients with RVH and in 15%-20% of those with essential hypertension. Thus, an elevated PRA is of limited diagnostic significance and its absence in no way rules out RVH. However, the predictive value of a PRA may be enhanced if obtained 1 to 2 hours after the ingestion of 25-50 mg of captopril (done in conjunction with a renogram or not). However, the captopril test used to assess the PRA response is limited by several factors, including a confounding influence from concomitant antihypertensive medications, a reduction in accuracy in the presence of mild renal insufficiency, as well as difficulty in standardizing the test.

Duplex Ultrasonography

Duplex ultrasonography combines B-mode ultrasound and Doppler examination and is an excellent test to detect RAS. It is the least expensive of the imaging modalities and provides useful information about the degree of stenosis, kidney size, and other associated disease processes (e.g., aneurysms or obstruction). Duplex ultrasonography may also be useful in predicting patients who will demonstrate an improvement in BP control or renal function after renal artery angioplasty and stenting. Despite these advantages, the utility of duplex Doppler ultrasonography as a screening tool is limited because it is time-consuming, operator dependent, and technically difficult to perform. In addition, intrarenal vascular lesions and multiple (and even main) renal arteries may be missed, particularly in obese patients or in those with overlying intestinal gas.

Magnetic Resonance Imaging

Magnetic resonance angiography (MRA) provides excellent imaging of the abdominal vasculature and associated anatomical structures. Contrast-enhanced MRA provides a superior quality study when compared with noncontrast studies. Gadolinium chelate is the contrast agent of choice and, unlike ionic and nonionic iodinated contrast agents, it is not nephrotoxic and can be used safely in patients with renal insufficiency. However, the visualization of distal, intrarenal, and accessory renal arteries that may have hemodynamically significant occlusive lesions remains suboptimal. MRA can also noninvasively determine both the absolute renal blood flow and the GFR and thus assess the functional significance of renovascular lesions. Patients with metallic implants, such as some mechanical heart valves, cerebral aneurysm clips, and electrically activated implants (e.g., pacemakers and spinal cord stimulators), cannot be studied by MRA. Most patients with IVC filters can be safely studied.

Angiography

Angiography, the gold standard for arterial imaging, is infrequently needed for the formal diagnosis of RAS. Angiography should be reserved for patients with an established diagnosis with indications to proceed with PTA and stenting. Renal angiography carries some risk, particularly of radiocontrast-induced acute renal failure or triggering atheroembolic disease. Gadolinium angiography is a non-nephrotoxic contrast agent that may be useful in patients with renal insufficiency. Renal vein PRA measurements are not useful screening tests for RAS. They seldom add value in shaping therapeutic decisions.

Because RAS is common in patients with coronary artery disease, some cardiologists perform an aortogram on the "way out" after completing a cardiac catheterization, which adds additional time and contrast to the procedure; moreover, the quality of such images is often suboptimal. Knowing that the patient has RAS adds nothing to the patient's overall management other than to entice the angiographer to stent the lesion in the absence of customary clinical indications. If the patient has an unambiguous indication for intervention (inability to control BP with a good antihypertensive regimen, diminishing renal function, or recurrent episodes of heart failure) and the clinician is prepared to perform angioplasty/stenting at a later date should significant RAS be found, then an aortogram at the time of cardiac catheterization is a sensible undertaking.

Selected Aspects of Treatment

Patients with normal renal function and atherosclerotic RAS that is focal, unilateral, and nonostial may be managed by angioplasty. Even though many patients with high-grade RAS remain stable for prolonged periods if BP is well controlled, surgical revascularization or PTRA with renal artery stenting may be needed to preserve renal function. Renal artery stenting has become an important adjunct to PTRA, being used to counteract elastic recoil and to offset the residual stenosis often observed after PTRA. Medical management is increasingly used in RAS patients with lesions not amenable to either angioplasty or surgery. Such patients typically require multiple medications. Diuretic therapy should be used cautiously to avoid volume contraction. ACE inhibitor or ARB therapy also should be used with care in patients with bilateral RAS. These drugs may be occasionally used in patients with unilateral RAS together with careful monitoring of renal function. Calcium-channel blockers remain an important component of therapy in patients with RAS.

Conclusion

Secondary hypertension can be insidious in its presentation and in many cases presents as refractory hypertension. A systematic approach to the refractory hypertensive might involve the steps shown in Table 10-2. Careful application of the principles cited in this table will many times decrease the number of cases of refractory hypertension and decrease the frequency with which diagnostic work-ups are considered for presumed secondary causes of hypertension.

Key Points

- Secondary hypertension is common in clinical practice if a broad definition is applied. A thorough history and physical exam with an emphasis on concomitant medications, alcohol intake, and over-the-counter medication use often provides important clues to the origin of secondary hypertension.

- Various patterns of secondary hypertension exist, including new-onset hypertension in a previously normotensive individual, loss of blood pressure control in a previously well-controlled patient, and/or labile blood pressure in the setting of either of these two patterns. Once a blood pressure pattern has been characterized it may provide useful information in sorting through possible secondary causes.

- Medication non-compliance is a frequent factor behind a lapse in blood pressure control. This may be one of the more difficult factors to establish in the course of patient management.

- Pseudoresistance in the form of tachycardia or subtle degrees of fluid retention (without edema) are common factors leading to antihypertensive medication resistance and should be considered before proceeding with a diagnostic work-up for secondary causes of hypertension.

- Endocrine forms of secondary hypertension, such as pheochromocytoma and Cushing's disease, are uncommon. Conversely, primary aldosteronism occurs with sufficient frequency to be considered in the resistant hypertensive. Primary aldosteronism can be insidious in its presentation because it is not always accompanied by hypokalemia.

- Sleep apnea, depression, and panic disorders are common and poorly appreciated secondary causes of hypertension. Thorough questioning of a patient or immediate family members often provides the basis for the diagnosis of these disorders.

BIBLIOGRAPHY

Arnaldi G, Angeli A, Atkinson AB, et al. Diagnosis and complications of Cushing's syndrome: a consensus statement. J Clin Endocrinol Metab. 2003;88:5593-602.

Brown MA, Buddle ML, Martin A. Is resistant hypertension really resistant? Am J Hypertens. 2001;14;1263-9.

Calhoun DA, Nishizaka MK, Zaman MA, et al. Hyperaldosteronism among black and white subjects with resistant hypertension. Hypertension. 2002;40:892-6.

Calhoun DA, Zaman MA, Nishizaka MK. Resistant hypertension. Curr Hypertens Rep. 2002;4:221-8.

Davies SJ, Jackson PR, Ramsay LE, Ghahramani P. Drug intolerance due to non-specific adverse effects related to psychiatric morbidity in hypertensive patients. Arch Int Med. 2003;163:592-600.

Goodfriend TL, Calhoun DA. Resistant hypertension, obesity, sleep apnea, and aldosterone: theory and therapy. Hypertension. 2004;43:1-7.

Johnson AG. NSAIDs and blood pressure: clinical importance for older patients. Drugs Aging. 1998;12:17-27.

Kudva YC, Sawka AM, Young WF Jr. Clinical review 164. The laboratory diagnosis of adrenal pheochromocytoma: the Mayo Clinic experience. J Clin Endocrinol Metab. 2003;88:4533-9.

Muxfeldt ES, Bloch KV, Nogueira AR, Salles GF. Twenty-four hour ambulatory blood pressure monitoring pattern of resistant hypertension. Blood Press Monit. 2003;8:181-5.

Safian RD, Textor SC. Renal artery stenosis. N Engl J Med. 2001;344:431-42.

Wolk R, Shamsuzzaman AS, Somers VK. Obesity, sleep apnea, and hypertension. Hypertension. 2003;42:1067-74.

Xin X, He J, Frontini MG, et al. Effects of alcohol reduction on blood pressure: a meta-analysis of randomized controlled trials. Hypertension. 2001;38:1112-7.

Young WF Jr. Mini-review: primary aldosteronism: changing concepts in diagnosis and treatment. Endocrinology. 2003;144:2208-13.

Zierler RE. Screening for renal artery stenosis: is it justified? Mayo Clinic Proc. 2002;77:307-8.

Zimmerman U, Kraus T, Himmerich H, et al. Epidemiology, implications and mechanisms underlying weight gain in psychiatric patients. J Psych Res. 2003;37: 193-220.

11

■ ■ ■

Controversies and Safety of Antihypertensive Medications

Ehud Grossman, MD

Franz H. Messerli, MD

T here is consensus that lowering blood pressure is safe and beneficial (1-5). However, there are still some controversies regarding the treatment of hypertension (Table 11-1). In this chapter we discuss some of the controversies and show what is clearly safe and what is still open for debate.

Diuretics

Numerous prospective studies attest to the safety and efficacy of diuretics in reducing morbidity and mortality in hypertensive patients (2,3). However, the safety of diuretics in diabetic hypertensive patients has been debated.

Twelve years ago Warram et al showed that in diabetic hypertensive patients the risk of cardiovascular mortality was 3.8-fold higher in those treated with diuretics than in untreated patients (6). In contrast, later prospective studies showed that diuretics reduced cardiovascular morbidity and mortality in elderly diabetic hypertensive patients (7-9). The old belief that diuretics may paradoxically increase cardiovascular morbidity and mortality can be considered with the recent evidence of clear benefit with diuretics by looking at the dose used. In the past, a high dose of diuretic was used, whereas in the more recent studies a low-dose diuretic with or without potassium-sparing agents was used.

It is well accepted that the low-dose diuretic is effective in lowering blood pressure with minimal side effects. Increasing the dose adds very little to the control of blood pressure, whereas it increases substantially the

---

Table 11-1   Controversial Issues in Antihypertensive Therapy

1. Do all antihypertensive drugs provide equal morbidity and mortality benefits?
2. Does the choice of the first-line agent matter?
3. Are all drugs in the same class providing equal benefits?
4. How low should blood pressure be reduced? Is there a J-shaped curve?
5. How should antihypertensive drugs be combined?
6. What is the long-term safety of antihypertensive drugs?
7. What is optimal antihypertensive therapy in acute cerebrovascular disease or coronary heart disease?

---

rate of side effects such as hypokalemia, hyponatremia, hyperuricemia, and hypercholesterolemia (10). Similarly, the risk of sudden cardiac death was low in diuretic users when the dose was low and a potassium-sparing agent was added (11). The rationale of adding a potassium-sparing agent to a thiazide is supported by the recent evidence that addition of aldosterone antagonists to optimal treatment reduces cardiovascular morbidity and mortality in patients with congestive heart failure (12,13). Thus, it seems that the controversy regarding the efficacy and safety of diuretics in hypertension has been resolved by using a low-dose diuretic with the option of adding a potassium-sparing agent.

There is still controversy concerning whether a diuretic should be the first drug of choice in most hypertensive patients. The Antihypertensive and Lipid-Lowering Treatment to Prevent Heart Attack Trial (ALLHAT) and the Second Australian National Blood Pressure Study (ANBP2) are the first completed trials comparing first-step treatment with a thiazide-type diuretic vs. an angiotensin-converting enzyme (ACE) inhibitor for morbidity and mortality outcomes (9,14). Unfortunately, each study came to a different conclusion. Comparison between the studies is erroneous because blood pressure control was not the same in the studies. In the ALLHAT study, systolic blood pressure (SBP) was reduced 2 mm Hg more in the diuretic group than in the ACE inhibitor group, and the diuretic advantage for stroke was explained to a substantial degree by the SBP difference (9). However, the advantages of diuretics for heart failure and combined cardiovascular disease could not be explained merely by the SBP difference. In the ANBP2 study, blood pressure levels at the end of the study were the same in the diuretic and ACE inhibitors arms (14).

The difference in blood pressure control between the treatment arms in the two studies could not explain entirely the different results. Conceivably, the different results may be explained by the selection of the thiazides (chlorthalidone in the ALLHAT and hydrochlorothiazide in the ANBP) and the ACE inhibitors (lisinopril in the ALLHAT and enalapril in the ANBP study). It is interesting in this regard that in the MRFIT study there was a change in protocol after 5 years because in the clinics where patients received chlorthalidone, the outcome was better than in the ones where patients received hydrochlorothiazide (15). The authors argued in retrospect that this switch in the diuretic treatment may have explained the favorable outcome of those who were randomized to the special intervention program in the MRFIT study. The ALLHAT and ANBP2 studies also differed in racial distribution, in blinding, and in sample size or, what is most relevant, in the number of morbid events observed. Thus, the question is still open whether chlorthalidone is better than hydrochlorothiazide, or enalapril is better than lisinopril, or whether the agents of the same classes are similar and a diuretic may be superior to an ACE inhibitor only in a specific population.

Data from other studies, such as the STOP 2 and CAPPP, cannot solve this question because in the "conventional" arm clinicians were given free choice of starting with a diuretic or a beta-blocker (16,17). There is little question as to the safety and efficacy of a low-dose diuretic with a potassium-sparing agent in hypertension and in diabetes-hypertension. This does not mean, however, that thiazide diuretics should be the preferred agents in most patients. This controversy is reflected by the diametrically different approach presented by the recent American and European hypertension guidelines (18,19).

Beta-Blockers

Until the recent publication of the JNC-7, diuretics and beta-blockers were both recommended as the drug of choice for essential hypertension (20). Some indirect evidence suggests that beta-blockers may have benefits in middle-aged and younger patients (21-23). Although numerous epidemiologic studies attest to the safety and efficacy of diuretics in this regard, the data for beta-blockers are sketchy and unconvincing. In fact, the available data suggest that clinical benefits of beta-blockers are poorly documented and that beta-blockers may be inefficacious in the elderly, who account for a large segment of the hypertensive population (24). Monotherapy with a beta-blocker in the elderly does not reduce morbidity and mortality compared with placebo. The British Medical Research Council (MRC)-2 trial, a randomized, placebo controlled, single blinded study in patients aged 65 to 74 years, clearly documented that although blood pressure was lowered effectively by the cardioselective beta-blocker atenolol, morbidity and mortality of the beta-blocker group did not differ from that of the placebo group (3).

Moreover, patients who received the combination of beta-blockers and diuretics fared consistently worse than those receiving diuretics alone (25). In a recent meta-analysis, we showed that beta-blocker-based therapy does not reduce cardiovascular disease, coronary heart disease, or total mortality in elderly hypertensive patients (24). The recent LIFE study showed that atenolol-based therapy is inferior to losartan-based therapy in elderly hypertensive patients with ECG-documented left ventricular hypertrophy (26,27). Thus, despite their having a "beneficial" effect on the surrogate end point, i.e., blood pressure, beta-blocker therapy failed to favorably affect the real end point, i.e., heart attack, strokes, and sudden death in elderly patients.

Similarly, in a large case-control study, the risk of sudden cardiac death was distinctly higher in elderly patients receiving either beta-blocker as monotherapy or in combination with a thiazide diuretic than in patients receiving other therapy (calcium antagonists, ACE inhibitors, potassium-sparing diuretics) (28). This would indicate that beta-blocker therapy does needlessly expose millions of elderly hypertensive patients to adverse effects and cost while not conferring any benefit whatsoever. In all studies in the geriatric population in which beta-blockers were implied to reduce morbidity and mortality, they were used in combination with a diuretic (1,2,29,30). Thus, in the Swedish STOP trial, more than two thirds of the patients were receiving combination therapy, and no information was available regarding the effects of beta-blocker monotherapy (1). In the SHEP study, only 32% of patients were receiving atenolol (or reserpine), all of these in combination with a diuretic (2).

A sub-analysis by Kostis et al did not identify any additional benefits attributable to atenolol (or reserpine) that were independent of the ones conferred by the diuretic (29). In the study of Coope and Warrender, which demonstrated a significant reduction in the rate of strokes, 70% of patients in the treatment group were receiving atenolol and 60% were receiving bendrofluazide (30). None of these studies indicates that a beta-blocker alone or as an addition to the diuretic regimen significantly or independently affects morbidity and mortality.

In middle-aged and younger patients, a meta-analysis analyzing the three studies showed a decrease in total cardiovascular mortality in men of 14% and an increase in women of 16% in the beta-blocker group when compared with non-beta-blocker treatment (31). Thus, there is still a controversy regarding whether a beta-blocker should be considered as one of the first drugs of choice for hypertension in elderly patients.

The use of beta-blockers is even more of a question in diabetic hypertensive patients. The National High Blood Pressure Education Program Working Group recommended in 1994 to avoid beta-blockers in diabetic hypertensive patients because they can adversely affect peripheral blood flow and mask symptoms of hypoglycemia (32).

The class of the beta-blockers is heterogeneous, and it has been debated whether all the drugs in the class are the same. The recent Carvedilol or Metoprolol European Trial (COMET) study showed a superiority of carvedilol over metoprolol in patients with congestive heart failure (33). Both carvedilol and metoprolol have nonetheless been shown to significantly decrease mortality in those with congestive heart failure. However, the design of the study does not allow one to conclude that carvedilol is superior because blood pressure levels were lower in the carvedilol-treated group and metoprolol was used in a sub-therapeutic dose. This controversy still exists, and only a well-designed head-to-head comparative study with two beta-blockers will be able to resolve the uncertainty.

Calcium Channel Bockers

Calcium channel blockers (CCBs) are widely used as antihypertensive agents. Physicians and patients like them because of their efficacy, metabolic neutrality, and clean side-effect profile. Several years ago a plethora of publications showed that hypertensive patients treated with short-acting CCBs are at increased risk for myocardial infarction and have a higher mortality rate compared with patients treated with other anti-hypertensive drugs, and CCBs have been accused of increasing the risk of cancer among hypertensive patients (34-39). These studies were uncritically extrapolated to all CCBs as a class, and they cast doubt on their safety and efficacy, alarmed patients, and frustrated physicians. However, recent prospective randomized studies attested to the safety of CCBs (9,16,40-42). They showed clearly that these agents are beneficial in reducing cardiovascular morbidity and mortality (4,9,16,40,41,43). CCBs are less effective than diuretics and ACE inhibitors in preventing congestive heart failure and less effective than blockers of the renin angiotensin system in preventing renal failure, but they are as effective as the renin angiotensin system blockers in reducing cardiovascular morbidity and mortality (9,16,41,43-46).

The risk of stroke or any cardiovascular event is almost doubled in hypertensive patients with diabetes mellitus (47). Lowering blood pressure markedly decreases the rate of cardiovascular events and renal deterioration in these patients (42,48-50). A few years ago two studies showed that CCBs are less effective than ACE inhibitors in preventing cardiovascular events in diabetic hypertensive patients (51,52). These results cast doubt on the safety and efficacy of CCBs in diabetic hypertensive patients. However, the recent results from the Syst-Eur, INSIGHT, and ALLHAT studies (8,9,53) showed that CCBs reduce cardiovascular morbidity and mortality in diabetic hypertensive patients. We recently showed that CCBs are as effective as diuretics and ACE inhibitors in reducing cardiovascular morbidity and mortality in diabetic hypertensive patients (54). Thus, it seems that CCBs are less effective than other agents in preventing congestive heart failure and renal deterioration, but they are safe and clearly reduce cardiovascular morbidity and mortality in hypertensive patients with or without diabetes mellitus.

Angiotensin-Converting Enzyme Inhibitors

Angiotensin-converting enzyme (ACE) inhibitors became very popular in the treatment of hypertension because, in addition to lowering blood pressure, they prolong life in patients with congestive heart failure, they prevent renal deterioration in patients with diabetic nephropathy and with nondiabetic renal failure, and they reduce morbidity and mortality in high-risk patients (44,55-68). Despite their advantages in subgroups of patients, they were not superior to other agents in prospective randomized trials in hypertensive patients (9,16,17,69). Surprisingly, in the CAPPP and ALLHAT studies, ACE inhibitors were even less effective than the conventional therapy or diuretic in preventing first stroke (9,17). In the recent PROGRESS trial in patients with cerebrovascular disease, combination therapy of a diuretic (indapamide) and ACE inhibitor (perindopril) reduced the risk of stroke by 43% when compared with placebo (70). However, perindopril alone, despite lowering systolic blood pressure by 5 mm Hg, decreased stroke risk only by a non-significant 5%.

It is possible that the benefit observed in high-risk patients was related to blood pressure reduction, and not to the specific effect of ACE inhibition (71). This assumption is supported by the observation of Svensson et al that the mild blood pressure fall observed in the clinic in the ramipril-treated group of the HOPE study underestimated the true blood pressure fall (72). Nevertheless, despite the controversy whether the beneficial effects of ACE inhibitors are related to blood pressure reduction or to the intrinsic effect of ACE inhibition, it seems safe to recommend ACE inhibitors to many hypertensive patients. It should be noted that most patients benefit from the combination of an ACE inhibitor and a diuretic.

Angiotensin-Receptor Blockers

Blocking the renin angiotensin aldosterone system (RAAS) with ACE inhibitors reduces cardiovascular morbidity and mortality in patients with high cardiovascular risk (67,68). Moreover, ACE inhibitors reduce the risk of recurrent stroke in patients with a history of stroke or transient ischemic attack (70). However, ACE inhibitors enhance prostaglandin synthesis and decrease the degradation of bradykinin (73,74), which may be responsible for their adverse effects. An alternative way to block the RAAS is by the new class of drugs, the angiotensin II (AII) receptor blockers (ARBs), which block AII activity at the receptor site. This class has been shown to be safe, well tolerated, and effective for blood pressure control in young and elderly patients (75-77). Recently, several studies showed that this class of drugs confers renal benefits in patients with diabetic nephropathy (45,78), reduces the rate of stroke in hypertensive patients better than the conventional treatment (26,27,79), and is effective in patients with congestive heart failure (80-86).

However, it is controversial whether ARBs are better at protecting the kidney than ACE inhibitors in patients with type 2 diabetes mellitus, and whether they reduce the risk of stroke better than ACE inhibitors. ARBs and

ACE inhibitors were not compared, so it remains only speculation that ARBs should be the drug of choice in these conditions. One should keep in mind that most diabetic patients are dying of cardiovascular events rather than of renal failure, and, because ACE inhibitors have been shown to reduce cardiovascular morbidity and mortality in these patients, they may be a better initial choice than ARBs in diabetic patients (66). This controversy still holds after the recent published studies, and it seems that ARBs may be a substitute or an additional but not superior therapy to ACE inhibitors (80,82,85,87-89).

Alpha-Blockers

Alpha blockers had great promise in the treatment of hypertension because, in addition to lowering blood pressure, they improve insulin resistance and lipid profile (90,91). However, the recent results of the ALLHAT study showed that alpha-blockers are less effective than diuretics in preventing cardiovascular events, mainly heart failure (92,93). Because of these results, the National Institutes of Health recommended not to use an alpha-blocker as the first drug of choice in hypertension. It is noteworthy that the systolic blood pressure was higher by 2 mm Hg in the doxazosin-treated patients than in the diuretic-treated patients, and the high rate of heart failure began very shortly after randomization (92). The ALLHAT results with the ACE inhibitor were similar to the results with alpha-blockers, but the ACE inhibitor remained a safe and effective first choice in hypertensive patients (9). Thus, although an alpha-blocker seems to be a safe antihypertensive agent, because of the ALLHAT results it should not be used as the first antihypertensive drug, just as an add-on therapy.

The Importance of Metabolic Neutrality of Antihypertensive Agents

Recent prospective studies have shown that the rate of developing diabetes mellitus is different with various drugs. Treatment with ACE inhibitors may reduce the rate of new-onset diabetes mellitus. In the HOPE study, the risk of developing diabetes mellitus was 34% less in patients treated with ramipril than in those not treated with ramipril (94). In the recent ALLHAT study, the rate of new-onset diabetes mellitus was higher with diuretic treatment (11.6%) than with either calcium antagonist (9.8%) or ACE inhibitor (8.1%) (9). The impact of the higher rate of developing diabetes mellitus with diuretic either alone or in combination with a beta-blocker is unclear. In the ALLHAT study despite the high rate of new-onset diabetes mellitus with diuretic, this treatment exerted the greatest benefit (9). Similarly, in the UKPDS, treatment with beta-blocker increased fasting plasma glucose levels but still gave maximal benefit (69). However, clinical experience teaches us that long-term follow-up of many years is required to uncover the potential harm of diuretics in regard to the higher rate of new-onset diabetes mellitus. Alternatively, it is possible that lowering blood pressure is the most important target of treatment, and drugs that lower blood pressure, even if they impair glucose metabolism, are effective in reducing morbidity and mortality. This issue is a matter of controversy that may be resolved when data from very long-term follow-up studies are available.

Long-Term Safety of Antihypertensive Therapy

Most prospective randomized trials last 4 to 6 years and therefore provide little if any information about long-term safety of antihypertensive drug classes. Many patients are exposed to blood pressure–lowering drugs for many decades, and drug induced changes could be cumulative. This is potentially true with the adverse metabolic effects that are seen with the diuretics and the beta-blockers. Clearly, the increased risk of new-onset diabetes with these drugs, alone or in combination, will not translate into increased morbidity and mortality in a study lasting only 4-6 years (9). After decades, however, sustained diabetes may have an important impact on cardiovascular morbidity and mortality. The same reasoning holds true for carcinogenicity of antihypertensive drugs. Recently, we have documented that long-term treatment with thiazide diuretics is a low-grade risk for renal cell carcinoma (95). The risk is higher in women than in men and seems to increase in parallel with the duration of diuretic exposure. Again, this risk of carcinogenicity is unlikely to be discovered in short-term (4-6 years) prospective, randomized trials because, similar to other carcinogenic substances such as tobacco, the exposure needed exceeds 2 decades. Diuretics have the longest track record of any antihypertensive drug class and, therefore, have been intensively scrutinized. Little, if anything, should be concluded about long-term safety, particularly with regard to carcinogenicity of other antihypertensive drug classes.

Combination Therapy

Numerous trials have been designed to provide a head-to-head comparison of two antihypertensive drugs. In most of these trials, add-on therapy was used in both therapeutic arms. However, there is little information regarding whether add-on therapy to lower blood pressure reduces morbidity and mortality. In the MRC trial in the elderly, the addition of a beta-blocker to the thiazide diuretic distinctly diminished the benefits (cardiovascular morbidity and mortality), and the benefits disappeared completely with beta-blocker monotherapy. Similarly, in the SHEP trial the addition of a beta-blocker did not provide any further benefits despite the initial fall in arterial pressure (29). Given that more than two-thirds of patients with stage I and stage II hypertension will need combination therapy, we urgently need studies allowing us to assess the benefits of one combination versus another.

■ ■ ■

Key Points

- There is general consensus that lowering blood pressure is safe and beneficial; however, there are still some controversies pertaining to the treatment of hypertension.

- Diuretics have been shown to increase the risk of new-onset diabetes and should not be used as first-line drugs in patients at risk.

- Beta-blockers have never been shown to reduce morbidity and mortality in elderly patients with hypertension; their monotherapeutic use should be avoided in uncomplicated elderly hypertensive patients.

- Calcium antagonists are safe and efficacious for the treatment of hypertension.

- Blockers of the renin angiotensin system (ACE inhibitors, ARBs) may have a particular advantage in patients with congestive heart failure and diabetic hypertensive renal disease.

- Long-term safety is not well documented for most antihypertensive drug classes; diuretics have been shown to confer a low-grade risk of renal cell carcinoma.

■ ■ ■

REFERERNCES

1. **Dahlof B, Lindholm LH, Hansson L, et al.** Morbidity and mortality in the Swedish Trial in Old Patients with Hypertension (STOP-Hypertension). Lancet. 1991;338:1281-5.

2. **SHEP Cooperative Research Group.** Prevention of stroke by antihypertensive drug treatment in older persons with isolated systolic hypertension. JAMA. 1991; 265:3255-64.

3. **Medical Research Council Working Party.** MRC trial of treatment of hypertension in older adults: principal results. BMJ. 1992;304:405-12.

4. **Staessen JA, Fagard R, Thijs L, et al.** Randomised double-blind comparison of placebo and active treatment for older patients with isolated systolic hypertension. Lancet. 1997;350:757-64.

5. **Staessen JA, Wang JG, Thijs L.** Cardiovascular protection and blood pressure reduction: a meta-analysis. Lancet. 2001;358:1305-15.

6. **Warram JH, Laffel LM, Valsania P, et al.** Excess mortality associated with diuretic therapy in diabetes mellitus. Arch Intern Med. 1991;151:1350-6.

7. **Curb JD, Pressel SL, Cutler JA, et al.** Effect of diuretic-based antihypertensive treatment on cardiovascular disease risk in older diabetic patients with isolated systolic hypertension. JAMA. 1996;276:1886-92.

8. **Mancia G, Brown M, Castaigne A, et al.** Outcomes with nifedipine GITS or Co-amilozide in hypertensive diabetics and nondiabetics in Intervention as a Goal in Hypertension (INSIGHT). Hypertension. 2003;41:431-6.

9. **ALLHAT Officers and Coordinators for the ALLHAT Collaborative Research Group.** The Antihypertensive and Lipid-Lowering Treatment to Prevent Heart Attack Trial. Major outcomes in high-risk hypertensive patients randomized to angiotensin-converting enzyme inhibitor or calcium channel blocker vs diuretic. JAMA. 2002;288:2981-97.

10. **Carlsen JE, Kober L, Torp-Pedersen C, Johansen P.** Relation between dose of bendrofluazide, antihypertensive effect, and adverse biochemical effects. BMJ. 1990;300:975-8.

11. **Siscovick DS, Raghunathan TE, Psaty BM, et al.** Diuretic therapy for hypertension and the risk of primary cardiac arrest. N Engl J Med. 1994;330:1852-7.

12. **Pitt B, Remme W, Zannad F, et al.** Eplerenone, a selective aldosterone blocker, in patients with left ventricular dysfunction after myocardial infarction. N Engl J Med. 2003;348:1309-21.

13. **Pitt B, Zannad F, Remme WJ, et al.** The effect of spironolactone on morbidity and mortality in patients with severe heart failure. N Engl J Med. 1999;341:709-17.

14. **Wing LM, Reid CM, Ryan P, et al.** A comparison of outcomes with angiotensin-converting enzyme inhibitors and diuretics for hypertension in the elderly. N Engl J Med. 2003;348:583-92.

15. Mortality after 10½ years for hypertensive participants in the Multiple Risk Factor Intervention Trial. Circulation. 1990;82:1616-28.

16. **Hansson L, Lindholm LH, Ekbom T, et al.** Randomised trial of old and new antihypertensive drugs in elderly patients: cardiovascular mortality and morbidity the Swedish Trial in Old Patients with Hypertension-2 study. Lancet. 1999;354:1751-6.

17. **Hansson L, Lindholm LH, Niskanen L, et al.** Effect of angiotensin-converting-enzyme inhibition compared with conventional therapy on cardiovascular morbidity and mortality in hypertension. Lancet. 1999;353:611-6.

18. **Guidelines Committee.** 2003 European Society of Hypertension-European Society of Cardiology guidelines for the management of arterial hypertension. J Hypertens. 2003;21:1011-53.

19. **Chobanian AV, Bakris GL, Black HR, et al.** The Seventh Report of the Joint National Committee on Prevention, Detection, Evaluation, and Treatment of High Blood Pressure: the JNC-7 report. JAMA. 2003;289:2560-72.

20. The Sixth Report of the Joint National Committee on Prevention, Detection, Evaluation, and Treatment of High Blood Pressure. Arch Intern Med. 1997;157:2413-46.

21. **Medical Research Council Working Party.** MRC trial of treatment of mild hypertension: principal results. BMJ. 1985;291:97-104.

22. **The IPPPSH Collaborative Group.** Cardiovascular risk and risk factors in a randomized trial of treatment based on the beta-blocker oxprenolol. J Hypertens. 1985;3:379-92.

23. **Wilhelmsen L, Berglund G, Elmfeldt D, et al.** Beta-blockers versus diuretics in hypertensive men: main results from the HAPPHY trial. J Hypertens. 1987;5:561-72.

24. **Messerli FH, Grossman E, Goldbourt U.** Are beta-blockers efficacious as first-line therapy for hypertension in the elderly? JAMA. 1998;279:1903-7.

25. **Lever AF, Brennan PJ.** MRC trial of treatment in elderly hypertensives. Clin Exp Hypertens. 1993;15:941-52.

26. **Dahlof B, Devereux RB, Kjeldsen SE, et al.** Cardiovascular morbidity and mortality in the Losartan Intervention For Endpoint reduction in hypertension study (LIFE): a randomised trial against atenolol. Lancet. 2002;359:995-1003.

27. **Lindholm LH, Ibsen H, Dahlof B, et al.** Cardiovascular morbidity and mortality in patients with diabetes in the Losartan Intervention for Endpoint Reduction in Hypertension Study: a randomised trial against atenolol. Lancet. 2002;359:1004-10.

28. **Hoes AW, Grobbee DE, Lubsen J, et al.** Diuretics, beta-blockers, and the risk for sudden cardiac death in hypertensive patients. Ann Intern Med. 1995;123:481-7.

29. **Kostis JB, Berge KG, Davis BR, et al.** Effect of atenolol and reserpine on selected events in the systolic hypertension in the elderly program (SHEP). Am J Hypertens. 1995;8:1147-53.

30. **Coope J, Warrender TS.** Randomised trial of treatment of hypertension in elderly patients in primary care. BMJ. 1986;293:1145-51.

31. Primary prevention with metoprolol in patients with hypertension (letter). JAMA. 1988;260:1713-6.

32. **National High Blood Pressure Education Program Working Group.** Report on hypertension in diabetes. Hypertension. 1994;23:145-58; discussion 159-60.

33. **Poole-Wilson PA, Swedberg K, Cleland JG, et al.** Comparison of carvedilol and metoprolol on clinical outcomes in patients with chronic heart failure in the Carvedilol or Metoprolol European Trial (COMET). Lancet. 2003;362:7-13.

34. **Pahor M, Guralnik JM, Corti MC, et al.** Long-term survival and use of antihypertensive medications in older persons. J Am Geriatr Soc. 1995;43:1191-7.

35. **Borhani NO, Mercuri M, Borhani PA, et al.** Final outcome results of the Multicenter Isradipine Diuretic Atherosclerosis Study (MIDAS). JAMA. 1996;276:785-91.

36. **Furberg CD, Psaty BM, Meyer JV.** Nifedipine: dose-related increase in mortality in patients with coronary heart disease. Circulation. 1995;92:1326-31.

37. **Psaty BM, Heckbert SR, Koepsell TD, et al.** The risk of myocardial infarction associated with antihypertensive drug therapies. JAMA. 1995;274:620-5.

38. **Pahor M, Guralnik JM, Salive ME, et al.** Do calcium channel blockers increase the risk of cancer? Am J Hypertens. 1996;9:695-9.

39. **Fitzpatrick AL, Daling JR, Furberg CD, et al.** Use of calcium channel blockers and breast carcinoma risk in postmenopausal women. Cancer. 1997;80:1438-47.

40. **Lindholm LH, Anderson H, Ekbom T, et al.** Relation between drug treatment and cancer in hypertensives in the Swedish Trial in Old Patients with Hypertension 2: a 5-year, prospective, randomised, controlled trial. Lancet. 2001;358:539-44.

41. **Brown MJ, Palmer CR, Castaigne A, et al.** Morbidity and mortality in patients randomised to double-blind treatment with a long-acting calcium-channel blocker or diuretic in the International Nifedipine GITS study. Lancet. 2000;356:366-72.

42. **Hansson L, Zanchetti A, Carruthers SG, et al.** Effects of intensive blood-pressure lowering and low-dose aspirin in patients with hypertension: principal results of the Hypertension Optimal Treatment (HOT) randomised trial. Lancet. 1998;351:1755-62.

43. **Hansson L, Hedner T, Lund-Johansen P, et al.** Randomised trial of effects of calcium antagonists compared with diuretics and beta-blockers on cardiovascular morbidity and mortality in hypertension: the Nordic Diltiazem (NORDIL) study. Lancet. 2000;356:359-65.

44. **Agodoa LY, Appel L, Bakris GL, et al.** Effect of ramipril vs amlodipine on renal outcomes in hypertensive nephrosclerosis: a randomized controlled trial. JAMA. 2001;285:2719-28.

45. **Lewis EJ, Hunsicker LG, Clarke WR, et al.** Renoprotective effect of the angiotensin-receptor antagonist irbesartan in patients with nephropathy due to type 2 diabetes. N Engl J Med. 2001;345:851-60.

46. **Berl T, Hunsicker LG, Lewis JB, et al.** Cardiovascular outcomes in the Irbesartan Diabetic Nephropathy Trial of patients with type 2 diabetes and overt nephropathy. Ann Intern Med. 2003;138:542-9.

47. **Grossman E, Messerli FH, Goldbourt U.** High blood pressure and diabetes mellitus: are all antihypertensive drugs created equal? Arch Intern Med. 2000;160:2447-52.

48. **Parving HH, Smidt UM.** Hypotensive therapy reduces microvascular albumin leakage in insulin-dependent diabetic patients with nephropathy. Diabet Med. 1986;3:312-5.

49. **Parving HH, Andersen AR, Smidt UM, Svendsen PA.** Early aggressive antihypertensive treatment reduces rate of decline in kidney function in diabetic nephropathy. Lancet. 1983;1:1175-9.

50. **UK Prospective Diabetes Study Group.** Tight blood pressure control and risk of macrovascular and microvascular complications in type 2 diabetes. BMJ. 1998;317: 703-13.

51. **Estacio RO, Jeffers BW, Hiatt WR, et al.** The effect of nisoldipine as compared with enalapril on cardiovascular outcomes in patients with non-insulin-dependent diabetes and hypertension. N Engl J Med. 1998;338:645-52.

52. **Tatti P, Pahor M, Byington RP, et al.** Outcome results of the Fosinopril Versus Amlodipine Cardiovascular Events Randomized Trial (FACET) in patients with hypertension and NIDDM. Diabetes Care. 1998;21:597-603.

53. **Tuomilehto J, Rastenyte D, Birkenhager WH, et al.** Effects of calcium-channel blockade in older patients with diabetes and systolic hypertension. N Engl J Med. 1999;340:677-84.

54. **Grossman E, Messerli FH.** Are calcium antagonists beneficial in diabetic patients with hypertension? Am J Med. 2004;116:44-9.

55. **Pfeffer MA, Braunwald E, Moye LA, et al.** Effect of captopril on mortality and morbidity in patients with left ventricular dysfunction after myocardial infarction. Results of the survival and ventricular enlargement trial. N Engl J Med. 1992;327:669-77.

56. **Pfeffer MA, Lamas GA, Vaughan DE, et al.** Effect of captopril on progressive ventricular dilatation after anterior myocardial infarction. N Engl J Med. 1988;319:80-6.

57. Effects of enalapril on mortality in severe congestive heart failure. Results of the Cooperative North Scandinavian Enalapril Survival Study (CONSENSUS). N Engl J Med. 1987;316:1429-35.

58. **The SOLVD Investigators.** Effect of enalapril on survival in patients with reduced left ventricular ejection fractions and congestive heart failure. N Engl J Med. 1991;325:293-302.

59. **The Acute Infarction Ramipril Efficacy Study Investigators.** Effect of ramipril on mortality and morbidity of survivors of acute myocardial infarction with clinical evidence of heart failure. Lancet. 1993;342:821-8.

60. **Viberti G, Mogensen CE, Groop LC, Pauls JF.** Effect of captopril on progression to clinical proteinuria in patients with insulin-dependent diabetes mellitus and microalbuminuria. JAMA. 1994;271:275-9.

61. **Lewis EJ, Hunsicker LG, Bain RP, Rohde RD.** The effect of angiotensin-converting-enzyme inhibition on diabetic nephropathy. N Engl J Med. 1993;329:1456-62.

62. **Ruggenenti P, Perna A, Gherardi G, et al.** Renoprotective properties of ACE-inhibition in non-diabetic nephropathies with non-nephrotic proteinuria. Lancet. 1999;354:359-64.

63. **Ruggenenti P, Perna A, Gherardi G, et al.** Renal function and requirement for dialysis in chronic nephropathy patients on long-term ramipril: REIN follow-up trial. Lancet. 1998;352:1252-6.

64. **The GISEN Group.** Randomised placebo-controlled trial of effect of ramipril on decline in glomerular filtration rate and risk of terminal renal failure in proteinuric, non-diabetic nephropathy. Lancet. 1997;349:1857-63.

65. **Ravid M, Savin H, Jutrin I, et al.** Long-term stabilizing effect of angiotensin-converting enzyme inhibition on plasma creatinine and on proteinuria in normotensive type II diabetic patients. Ann Intern Med. 1993;118:577-81.

66. **Heart Outcomes Prevention Evaluation Study Investigators.** Effects of ramipril on cardiovascular and microvascular outcomes in people with diabetes mellitus: results of the HOPE study and MICRO-HOPE substudy. Lancet. 2000;355:253-9.

67. **Fox KM, EUROPA Investigators.** Efficacy of perindopril in reduction of cardiovascular events among patients with stable coronary artery disease: randomised, double-blind, placebo-controlled, multicentre trial. Lancet. 2003;362:782-8.

68. **Yusuf S, Sleight P, Pogue J, et al.** Effects of an angiotensin-converting-enzyme inhibitor, ramipril, on cardiovascular events in high-risk patients. N Engl J Med. 2000;342:145-53.

69. **UK Prospective Diabetes Study Group.** Efficacy of atenolol and captopril in reducing risk of macrovascular and microvascular complications in type 2 diabetes. BMJ. 1998;317:713-20.

70. **PROGRESS Collaborative Group.** Randomised trial of a perindopril-based blood-pressure-lowering regimen among 6105 individuals with previous stroke or transient ischaemic attack. Lancet. 2001;358:1033-41.

71. **Messerli FH, White WB, Staessen JA.** If only cardiologists did properly measure blood pressure: blood pressure recordings in daily practice and clinical trials. J Am Coll Cardiol. 2002;40:2201-3.

72. **Svensson P, de Faire U, Sleight P, et al.** Comparative effects of ramipril on ambulatory and office blood pressures: a HOPE Substudy. Hypertension. 2001;38:E28-32.

73. **Gavras I.** Bradykinin-mediated effects of ACE inhibition. Kidney Int. 1992;42:1020-9.

74. **Quilley J, Duchin KL, Hudes EM, McGiff JC.** The antihypertensive effect of captopril in essential hypertension: relationship to prostaglandins and the kallikrein-kinin system. J Hypertens. 1987;5:121-8.

75. **Gillis JC, Markham A.** Irbesartan. A review of its pharmacodynamic and pharmacokinetic properties and therapeutic use in the management of hypertension. Drugs. 1997;54:885-902.

76. **Goa KL, Wagstaff AJ.** Losartan potassium: a review of its pharmacology, clinical efficacy and tolerability in the management of hypertension. Drugs. 1996;51:820-45.

77. **Markham A, Goa KL.** Valsartan. A review of its pharmacology and therapeutic use in essential hypertension. Drugs. 1997;54:299-311.

78. **Brenner BM, Cooper ME, de Zeeuw D, et al.** Effects of losartan on renal and cardiovascular outcomes in patients with type 2 diabetes and nephropathy. N Engl J Med. 2001;345:861-9.

79. **Lithell H, Hansson L, Skoog I, et al.** The Study on Cognition and Prognosis in the Elderly (SCOPE): principal results of a randomized double-blind intervention trial. J Hypertens. 2003;21:875-86.

80. **Pitt B, Poole-Wilson PA, Segal R, et al.** Effect of losartan compared with captopril on mortality in patients with symptomatic heart failure: randomised trial: the Losartan Heart Failure Survival Study ELITE II. Lancet. 2000;355:1582-7.

81. **Maggioni AP, Anand I, Gottlieb SO, et al.** Effects of valsartan on morbidity and mortality in patients with heart failure not receiving angiotensin-converting enzyme inhibitors. J Am Coll Cardiol. 2002;40:1414-21.

82. **Cohn JN, Tognoni G.** A randomized trial of the angiotensin-receptor blocker valsartan in chronic heart failure. N Engl J Med. 2001;345:1667-75.

83. **Yusuf S, Pfeffer MA, Swedberg K, et al.** Effects of candesartan in patients with chronic heart failure and preserved left-ventricular ejection fraction: the CHARM-Preserved Trial. Lancet. 2003;362:777-81.

84. **Granger CB, McMurray JJ, Yusuf S, et al.** Effects of candesartan in patients with chronic heart failure and reduced left-ventricular systolic function intolerant to angiotensin-converting-enzyme inhibitors: the CHARM-Alternative trial. Lancet. 2003;362:772-6.

85. **McMurray JJ, Ostergren J, Swedberg K, et al.** Effects of candesartan in patients with chronic heart failure and reduced left-ventricular systolic function taking angiotensin-converting-enzyme inhibitors: the CHARM-Added trial. Lancet. 2003;362:767-71.

86. **Pfeffer MA, Swedberg K, Granger CB, et al.** Effects of candesartan on mortality and morbidity in patients with chronic heart failure: the CHARM-Overall programme. Lancet. 2003;362:759-66.

87. **Grossman E, Messerli FH, Neutel JM.** Angiotensin II receptor blockers: equal or preferred substitutes for ACE inhibitors? Arch Intern Med. 2000;160:1905-11.

88. **Dickstein K, Kjekshus J.** Effects of losartan and captopril on mortality and morbidity in high-risk patients after acute myocardial infarction: the OPTIMAAL randomised trial. Lancet. 2002;360:752-60.

89. **Nakao N, Yoshimura A, Morita H, et al.** Combination treatment of angiotensin-II receptor blocker and angiotensin-converting-enzyme inhibitor in non-diabetic renal disease: a randomised controlled trial. Lancet. 2003;361:117-24.

90. **Pool JL.** Effects of doxazosin on coronary heart disease risk factors in the hypertensive patient. Br J Clin Pract Suppl. 1994;74:8-12.

91. **Grimm RH Jr, Flack JM, Grandits GA, et al.** Long-term effects on plasma lipids of diet and drugs to treat hypertension. JAMA. 1996;275:1549-56.

92. **ALLHAT Collaborative Research Group.** Major cardiovascular events in hypertensive patients randomized to doxazosin vs chlorthalidone. JAMA. 2000;283:1967-75.

93. **Messerli FH.** Implications of discontinuation of doxazosin arm of ALLHAT. Lancet. 2000;355:863-4.

94. **Yusuf S, Gerstein H, Hoogwerf B, et al.** Ramipril and the development of diabetes. JAMA. 2001;286:1882-5.

95. **Grossman E, Messerli FH, Goldbourt U.** Does diuretic therapy increase the risk of renal cell carcinoma? Am J Cardiol. 1999;83:1090-3.

12

◾ ◾ ◾

Hypertensive Urgencies and Emergencies: Considerations for Treatment

C. Venkata S. Ram, MD

Various terms such as *crises, emergencies,* or *urgencies* have been used to describe acute complications of hypertension; they are all characterized by uncontrolled, severe, or abrupt hypertension resulting in acute serious and sometimes deadly cardiac, renal, or neurological complications. Hypertensive crises may occur with any type of hypertensive disorder. It is likely that any complication of hypertension (acute or chronic) is related to non-compliance and poor control of chronic hypertension. The true prevalence of hypertensive emergencies and urgencies is difficult to determine since the diagnostic criteria may vary from center to center. The diagnosis may also be imprecise as some physicians may (mis)classify headache or epistaxis or dizziness as a hypertensive urgency. The principal determinant of hypertensive crisis is the level of blood pressure rather than the cause of hypertension (1,2). In some clinical situations, such as sudden onset of hypertension in children with acute glomerulonephritis, toxemia of pregnancy, and drug-induced hypertension, the abruptness with which the blood pressure rises is more critical than the actual level of blood pressure. The complications of hypertensive crisis are largely reversible, if the treatment is rendered efficiently (3,4). In certain (but not all) clinical circumstances, immediate reduction of blood pressure is indicated, not because of its absolute level but because the coexisting complications may make any degree of hypertension dangerous. The risk/benefit ratio of immediate therapy in some forms of hypertensive crisis is not established.

Hypertensive crises are customarily categorized as either hypertensive emergencies or hypertensive urgencies (Tables 12-1 and 12-2). With hypertensive emergencies, the elevation in blood pressure causes immediate

---

Table 12-1   Examples of Hypertensive Emergencies

- Accelerated/malignant hypertension
- Hypertensive encephalopathy
- Acute left ventricular failure
- Acute aortic dissection
- Intracranial hemorrhage
- Pheochromocytoma crisis
- Monoamine oxidase inhibitor + tyramine interaction
- Eclampsia
- Substance/drug-induced acute hypertension

Table 12-2   Examples of Hypertensive Urgencies

- Accelerated/malignant hypertension*
- Severe hypertension associated with coronary artery disease
- Severe hypertension in the kidney transplant patient
- Preoperative hypertension
- Hypertension associated with burns

*Can also be considered as an emergency.

---

end-organ damage; hypertensive emergencies therefore carry poor prognosis unless the blood pressure level is reduced rather quickly (in a matter of a few hours). Hypertensive urgencies pose less immediate danger, and blood pressure should be reduced quickly, whereas in hypertensive urgencies, blood pressure reduction may be accomplished gradually (in several hours or days). There does not appear to be any arbitrary level of blood pressure that separates hypertensive emergencies from urgencies.

General Approach to a Patient with Hypertensive Emergency

The most critical decision in the management of hypertensive crises (emergencies or urgencies) is to assess the patient's clinical state and to ascertain whether the patient's condition truly needs emergency management. Patients with hypertensive emergencies should be hospitalized, and those with hypertensive urgencies may not always require prolonged hospital stay. The choice between oral and parenteral drug likewise depends on the clinical situation, whether it is a hypertensive emergency or urgency. The choice of parenteral drug is dictated by the clinical manifestations and concomitant medical problems associated with hypertensive crises (treatment of specific hypertensive crises is discussed later in this chapter). Although a secondary form of hypertension such as renal artery stenosis or adrenal hypertension may be a causative factor, the immediate goal should be to lower the blood pressure to a safe level instead of undertaking a diagnostic workup. The therapeutic premise underlying the management of hypertensive emergency is not only to lower the blood pressure quickly but to prevent, arrest, and reverse the target organ damage. Therefore, close supervision of the patient is mandatory while the blood pressure is being lowered. Hypertensive emergencies should be preferably managed in an intensive care unit to allow for continuous monitoring of the general hemodynamic status of the patient.

The level to which the blood pressure should be lowered varies with the type of hypertensive crisis and should be individualized; however, a reasonable goal for most hypertensive emergencies is to lower the diastolic blood pressure to 100 mm Hg (or to reduce the mean arterial pressure by 20%) over a period of minutes to hours. An important consideration in treating patients with hypertensive emergencies is the rapidity of onset and duration of action of the chosen drug.

Once the hypertensive emergency is resolved and the patient's clinical condition is stable, the physician should look into possible factors that might have contributed to the dangerous elevation of blood pressure, such as non adherence to prescribed therapy or the presence and/or progression of a secondary form of hypertension such as a renal artery stenosis or renal failure. After the patient's condition has been stabilized, the physician should discuss long-range and periodic outpatient follow-up plans; close follow-up is extremely important in these patients. Complications of therapy, mainly hypotension and ischemic brain damage, can occur in patients given multiple antihypertensive drugs in large doses without adequate monitoring (5). Gentle lowering of blood pressure, careful surveillance, and individualization of therapy can minimize such complications. Relatively asymptomatic patients who present with severe hypertension, that is, a diastolic blood pressure of 130 to 140 mm Hg, need not be treated with parenteral drugs. These patients should be managed on an individual basis, and the usual course would be to intensify or alter the previous antihypertensive therapy. All too often, asymptomatic patients or those without an acute problem are unnecessarily subjected to immediate therapy. Acute alteration of the level of the patient's blood pressure may be self-gratifying to the physician but is not indicated for most patients with asymptomatic severe hypertension. Indiscriminate use of therapeutic options such as nifedipine and furosemide should be strongly discouraged.

Parenteral Drugs for Hypertensive Emergencies

Parenteral drugs for rapid control of severe hypertension are listed in Table 12-3.

Sodium Nitroprusside

Sodium nitroprusside is a powerful antihypertensive useful for most hypertensive emergencies that possesses the property of rapid onset and offset

Table 12-3   Parenteral Drugs for Hypertensive Emergencies

Drug	Dose	Administration	Onset of Action	Duration of Action	Adverse Effects	Special Indications
Sodium nitroprusside	0.25-10 µg/kg/min	IV infusion	Within 30 sec	1-2 min	Hypotension, nausea, vomiting, muscle twitching, thiocyanide and cyanide intoxication, methemoglobinemia	Most hypertensive emergencies; caution with renal and hepatic insufficiency and high intracranial pressure
Fenoldopam	0.1-0.6 µg/kg/min	IV infusion	4-5 min	10-15 min	Reflex tachycardia, may rise intraocular pressure, headache, and nausea	Renal insufficiency, peri- and post-operative control of blood pressure
Glyceryl trinitrate	5-100 µg/min	IV infusion	2-5 min	3-5 min	Headache, nausea, vomiting, tolerance with prolonged use	Coronary insufficiency
Nicardipine	5-15 mg/h	IV infusion	5-10 min	1-4 h	Reflex tachycardia, headache, nausea, vomiting, flushing	Most hypertensive emergencies, caution with heart failure
Hydralazine	10-20 mg IV 10-50 mg IM	IV infusion	10-20 min	4-12 h	Reflex tachycardia, headache, nausea, vomiting, aggravation of angina	Eclampsia, caution with high intracranial pressure
Enalaprilat	1.25-5 mg every 6h	IV infusion	10-15 min	6-24 h	Hypotension, renal failure	Acute left ventricular failure
Labetalol	20-80 mg IV bolus every 10 min 2 mg/min infusion	IV bolus IV infusion	5 min	3-6 h	Nausea, vomiting, broncho-spasm, heart block, ortho-static hypotension	Most hypertensive emergencies except heart failure
Phentolamine	5-10 mg/min	IV bolus	1-2 min	3-5 min	Reflex tachycardia, headache	Pheochromocytoma

of action. The hypotensive response occurs within seconds after infusion is started and disappears almost as rapidly when the infusion is discontinued.

The initial infusion rate should be 0.3 ug/kg/min, which can be increased every 5 minutes until a desired blood pressure level is obtained. Once the desired effect of nitroprusside is achieved, the blood pressure should be continuously monitored. Hypotension is the most common adverse effect, but is avoidable. This agent should be avoided in patients with high intracranial pressure. Cyanide toxicity from nitroprusside, although extremely rare, has occurred. Prophylactic infusion of hydroxocobalamin (vitamin B) 25 mg/h, has been shown to decrease the cyanide concentration and tissue hypoxia resulting from nitroprusside infusion during surgery.

Thiocyanate toxicity secondary to nitroprusside is uncommon and occurs only with high doses and in the presence of renal failure. Treatment should be interrupted when the thiocyanate level is close to 10 mg/dL. Monitoring of plasma thiocyanate levels is not mandatory as long as the patient's clinical status is closely assessed. Treatment of thiocyanate toxicity requires discontinuation of the drug and institution of dialysis.

Intravenous Labetalol

Labetalol is a combined alpha- and beta-adrenergic blocking drug that can be used parenterally or orally for the treatment of hypertensive emergencies (oral labetalol is discussed later in this chapter). Intravenous labetalol administered as either a continuous infusion or bolus injections reduces the blood pressure promptly because of its rapid onset of action. Controlled smooth reduction in blood pressure may be obtained by continuous infusion of labetalol at the rate of 0.5 to 2 mg/min. As with nitroprusside, close monitoring of the patient is required during the infusion of labetalol therapy. Rapid (but not abrupt) lowering of blood pressure can also be accomplished with bolus injections of labetalol. Labetalol should not be used in patients who may have contraindication for use of beta-blockers such as heart failure, atrioventricular block, asthma, and chronic obstructive pulmonary disease.

Nicardipine Infusion

Nicardipine is a dihydropyridine calcium antagonist that exerts a prompt hemodynamic effect when given intravenously in patients with severe hypertension. Nicardipine infusion is started at 5.0 mg/h and can be titrated up gradually to obtain the desired therapeutic effect (6). Once a stable blood pressure level is reached, most patients do not require further dosage alterations. Thus, nicardipine pharmacodynamics resemble those of nitroprusside in terms of the onset, duration, and offset of action. Because of its mechanism of action (calcium channel blockade), nicardipine may be beneficial in preserving tissue perfusion. This property may be particularly advantageous in patients with ischemic disorders, coronary, cerebrovascular, and peripheral vascular disease. From my clinical experience with the use of nicardipine, I believe that it is a useful option in the management of severe hypertension with or without target organ damage.

Trimethaphan

Trimethaphan camsylate is a ganglion-blocking agent. It is the drug of choice for the medical treatment of acute aortic dissection. Like nitroprusside, trimethaphan should be administered as a continuous intravenous drip, and constant monitoring is necessary, preferably in the intensive care unit. The usual starting dose of the drug should be 1 mg/min titrated to obtain the desired blood pressure level. After prolonged infusion, tachyphylaxis may result from intravascular volume expansion, which can be partially overcome by effective diuretic therapy.

Hydralazine

The hypotensive action of hydralazine results from a direct relaxation of the vascular smooth muscle and is accompanied by reflex increases in stroke volume and heart rate, which can precipitate myocardial ischemia. Intramuscular or intravenous administration of hydralazine results in an unpredictable but definite fall in blood pressure. In the treatment of hypertensive emergencies, the initial dose should be 10 to 20 mg. The onset of the hypotensive effect occurs within 10 to 30 minutes, and its duration of action ranges from 3 to 9 hours. The dose and frequency of administration necessary to control the blood pressure are highly variable. The delayed onset and unpredictable degree of hypotensive effect present difficulties in titration. Nevertheless, hydralazine continues to be successfully employed in the treatment of eclampsia.

Phentolamine

Phentolamine, an alpha-receptor–blocking agent, is specifically indicated for treating hypertensive crises associated with increased circulating catecholamines, for example, pheochromocytoma crisis, certain cases of clonidine withdrawal syndrome, and crises resulting from monoamine oxidase inhibitor and drug-food interaction. The hypotensive effect of a single intravenous bolus injection is short lived and lasts less than 15 minutes. This drug may precipitate angina or cardiac arrhythmias.

Enalaprilat

Enalaprilat, by virtue of its mechanism of action, prevents conversion of angiotensin I to angiotensin II by blocking angiotensin-converting enzyme (ACE) and thus lowers the blood pressure. Enalaprilat is the only available parenteral ACE inhibitor. For hypertensive emergencies, it is given intravenously at a dosage ranging from 0.625 to 1.25 mg over 5 min and may be repeated every 6 hours. ACE inhibitors are contraindicated in patients with renal artery stenosis and in pregnant patients. ACE inhibitors can cause precipitous falls in blood pressure in patients who are hypovolemic. These drugs are especially valuable in treating hypertensive emergencies in patients with chronic heart failure.

Fenoldopam

Fenoldopam is a selective dopamine (DA_1) receptor agonist, which causes significant vasodilation. It is a short-acting parenteral arteriolar vasodilator, which lowers blood pressure by reducing peripheral vascular resistance (7,8). By the mode of its action on DA_1 receptor, fenoldopam causes remarkable renal vasodilation and promotes diuresis and natruresis (9). The half-life is estimated to be 5 minutes and the recommended starting dose is 0.1 µg/kg/min. Its onset of action is 5 minutes and maximum response is achieved within 15 minutes. The dose should be titrated to gradually attain the goal pressure. It can safely and effectively lower blood pressure in hypertensive emergencies and at the same time preserve or improve renal blood flow and cause natriuresis diuresis. Therefore, it may offer important advantages. My experience with fenoldopam in hypertensive emergencies has been gratifying (7). Comparative studies between nitroprusside and fenoldopam have shown that while both drugs are equally effective in reducing the blood pressure, fenoldopam offers important renal advantages over nitroprusside (10,11).

Nitroglycerin

Nitroglycerin is a weak systemic arterial dilator with a greater effect on large arteries than on smaller arteries. Low doses cause vasodilation; much higher doses are required to produce a fall in systemic blood pressure. Because of its pharmacologic actions, nitroglycerin infusion may be particularly beneficial in patients with coronary artery disease with or without hypertension. Nitroglycerin improves coronary perfusion. Although there are no controlled studies, nitroglycerin therapy can be considered in the management of severe hypertension associated with coronary artery disease. The usual initial dosage of nitroglycerin is 5 to 15 µg/min, and it is titrated upward to a desired therapeutic endpoint. It has a rapid onset (within 2-5 minutes) and offset of action. Although nitroglycerin has been used to achieve controlled hypotension, its main use continues to be in patients with unstable angina and acute myocardial infarction. Prolonged use may result in tolerance. Isosorbide dinitrate therapy has also been utilized for immediate treatment of severe hypertension, but its precise role and guidelines on how to use it are not fully delineated (12).

Diazoxide

Diazoxide has a direct relaxant effect on the vascular smooth muscle, causing a rapid fall in arterial blood pressure (13). The hypotensive effect of diazoxide is associated with striking increases in heart rate and cardiac output. Diazoxide produces a rapid fall in blood pressure within 1 minute, and the maximum effect is achieved within 2 to 5 minutes. The hypotensive effect of a single injection of diazoxide may last 2 to 15 hours, but if there is no effect from the first injection, an additional dose can be given within 30 minutes. Smaller bolus injections and slow intravenous infusions of diazoxide for the treatment of severe hypertension have been used, with the hope of reducing the dangers of drastic and precipitous reduction in blood pressure. The need to use diazoxide these days has been virtually eliminated by the availability of safe alternative drugs.

Transition from Parenteral to Oral Therapy

After the immediate management of a hypertensive emergency with parenteral therapy, oral agents should be initiated at the earliest opportunity. Generally, oral therapy can be begun while tapering off the parenteral drug. If possible, oral drugs should be started with a low dose, which can be increased gradually depending on the clinical response. It is important to detect and prevent postural hypotension during transition to oral therapy.

Role of Concomitant Diuretic Therapy

Diuretics per se have a limited role in the management of hypertensive emergencies; however, they potentiate the therapeutic response to nondiuretic agents. When the blood pressure does not respond satisfactorily to an adequate dose of the primary agent, adding a diuretic (furosemide) may be helpful. Certainly in volume overload states such as heart failure, concomitant administration of a loop diuretic is indicated for optimal results. Diuretics should not be used routinely in the management of hypertensive crises because previous volume depletion may be present in some conditions such as malignant hypertension. The need for diuretic therapy, therefore, should be individualized on the basis of the hemodynamic and renal function status of the patient.

Oral Drugs

Nifedipine

Nifedipine, a calcium channel blocker, given orally or sublingually, has been shown to reduce the blood pressure rapidly and has been found to be useful in the management of hypertensive crisis (14). Immediate reduction in blood pressure can be accomplished with sublingual (punctured capsule, or nifedipine liquid drawn out of the capsule with a syringe) or oral administration of the capsules. The drug is also effective when the capsule is bitten and then swallowed. The advantages of nifedipine are rapid onset of action and lack of central nervous system depression. It may cause reflex tachycardia. Because the duration of action of nifedipine is short, patients who receive this drug for hypertensive emergencies should be monitored for several hours to consider readministration of the drug. Abrupt fall in the blood pressure induced by nifedipine administration can cause certain adverse effects: symptomatic hypotension, tachycardia, and ischemic events. Therefore, the clinical need to use nifedipine capsules to lower the blood pressure urgently should be carefully assessed and avoided, if possible.

Clonidine

Clonidine therapy has been shown to produce an immediate antihypertensive effect with repetitive dosing. Typically, clonidine loading was accomplished in the emergency room by administering clonidine orally 0.1 mg every hour until the desired goal was obtained. Clonidine loading as therapy is on the decline because of the availability of safer and better-tolerated alternative therapies (discussed above), which do not cause drowsiness.

Angiotensin-Converting Enzyme Inhibitors

Captopril, an ACE inhibitor, has been found to be effective in the immediate treatment of severe hypertension and hypertensive crises. Captopril lowers the blood pressure promptly without causing tachycardia and, thus, offers a distinct hemodynamic advantage over direct arteriolar dilators; however, the maximal effect from orally administered captopril may not be attained for as long as 2 hours. On the other hand, there are some reports documenting the effectiveness of sublingual captopril in the treatment of hypertensive crisis (15). As experience with sublingual captopril is rather limited, further data have to be generated to define its role in the acute management of hypertensive crisis.

Minoxidil

Minoxidil is a powerful direct vasodilator and has been successfully used in the treatment of refractory or severe hypertension. Because of its relatively rapid onset of action and sustained duration, this drug has been used for the treatment of hypertensive crises. Minoxidil in doses ranging from 2.5 to 10 mg can be given every 4 to 6 hours initially in the treatment of severe hypertension. It works best when given along with a diuretic, and an adrenergic blocker is necessary to counteract the reflex tachycardia. Minoxidil should be used with caution in patients with acute coronary syndromes unless the patient is well beta-blocked.

Oral Labetalol

Labetalol, a combined alpha- and beta-adrenergic blocker, can be administered orally (100-300 mg) in the treatment of hypertensive urgencies. Because of its dual adrenergic blockade, the fall in blood pressure is not accompanied by reflex tachycardia, which can be beneficial especially in patients with coronary artery disease. Oral labetalol is effective within 1 to 3 hours and may be useful for hypertensive urgencies. But it has an unpredictable dose response and thus may not be ideal for acute situations. Labetalol is contra-indicated in patients with bronchospasm, heart block, significant bradycardia or heart failure.

Specific Hypertensive Emergencies and Their Treatment

Accelerated and Malignant Hypertension

Although the term "malignant" hypertension is used without a strict definition, the most striking characteristic of accelerated and malignant hypertension is the presence of acute vascular lesions in the kidney and in other target organs. Accelerated hypertension is clinically identified by the presence of severe retinopathy (without papilledema), exudates, hemorrhages, arteriolar narrowing, and spasm. Malignant hypertension, on the other hand, is considered an extension of the accelerated form and is characterized by the presence of papilledema. Both the accelerated and malignant forms of hypertension are associated with severe vascular injury to the kidney and other target organs. The manifestations of accelerated and malignant hypertension are listed in Table 12-4.

Clinical Manifestation and Diagnosis

The blood pressure level in malignant hypertension is usually quite high, with diastolic levels often in the range of 130 to 140 mm Hg, stage 2 hypertension (Table 12-5), but the degree of blood pressure elevation is an unreliable diagnostic criterion. It is the extent of vascular injury that determines the clinical manifestations. Severe headache, with or without coexisting encephalopathy, is a symptom. Often, the headache is occipital in location and may be more intense in the morning hours. Weight loss may occur in some patients with malignant hypertension as a result of initial natriuresis. Many patients with malignant hypertension report visual complaints ranging from blurring to blindness; drowsy feeling and altered mental status are

Table 12-4   Clinical Presentation of Accelerated and Malignant Hypertension

• Marked elevation of blood pressure	• Retinopathy
• Malaise; weight loss	• Renal failure (azotemia, proteinuria, hematuria, etc.)
• Headache	

Table 12-5   Blood Pressure Classification

	SBP, mm Hg		DBP, mm Hg
Normal	<120	*and*	<80
Pre-hypertension	120-139	*or*	80-89
Stage 1 hypertension	140-159	*or*	90-99
Stage 2 hypertension	≥160	*or*	≥100

Adapted from Chobanian AV, Bakris GL, Black HR, et al. JNC-7 Report. JAMA. 2003;289:2560-72; with permission.

common. Deterioration in these symptoms may indicate progression to en-cephalopathy or other cerebral complications. Congestive heart failure can be an occasional presenting feature of malignant hypertension as a direct consequence of left ventricular dysfunction or due to volume retention from concomitant renal failure. Azotemia, a common feature of malignant hypertension, may be associated with proteinuria. Renal function deterio-rates rapidly in many patients without appropriate therapeutic intervention. Even with treatment, renal function may decline at times due to reduced renal perfusion. Anemia is a common finding in malignant hypertension. The degree of anemia may give a clue as to the proximate cause: severe anemia suggests underlying chronic renal disease, whereas modest degrees may reflect microangiopathic hemolysis.

The diagnosis of accelerated and malignant hypertension can be best made clinically on the basis of history and clinical examination. Simple in-vestigations such as chest x-ray, electrocardiogram, complete blood count, blood urea nitrogen, creatinine, electrolytes, and urinalysis are sufficient for the preliminary management of malignant hypertension.

Treatment

Patients with accelerated and malignant hypertension should be treated in the hospital because the goal is not simply to lower the blood pressure but to stabilize, reverse target organ damages, and exclude reversible causes. Preferably, the patients should be treated in an intensive care unit; but in the absence of significant target organ dysfunction, they can be managed safely on the wards.

Although parenteral therapy is widely used in the initial treatment of malignant hypertension, various oral therapies can also be successfully used. ACE inhibitors, minoxidil, clonidine, prazosin, labetalol, and nifedip-ine have all been used for initial treatment of malignant hypertension, but there are no controlled prospective studies to offer precise guidelines on the preferred therapeutic options. The choice between oral and parenteral therapy depends on the monitoring facilities, condition of the patient, and coexisting complications. Once the blood pressure is brought to safe levels, appropriate oral therapy must be initiated based on the patient's renal, car-diac, and neurologic status.

Hypertensive Encephalopathy

Hypertensive encephalopathy is a serious and potentially lethal complica-tion of severe hypertension (4). Although hypertensive encephalopathy occurs mainly in patients with malignant hypertension, it can also result from sudden hypertension of short duration. Hypertensive encephalopathy carries a poor prognosis if not quickly recognized and treated. Hyper-tensive encephalopathy may be precipitated not only by elevation of blood pressure to severe levels in hypertensive patients, but also by the abrupt rise of blood pressure in previously normotensive individuals. So, hypertensive encephalopathy occurs more frequently when the hypertension is complicated by renal insufficiency than when the renal function is normal. The full clinical syndrome of hypertensive encephalopathy may take 12 to 48 hours to develop.

Clinical Manifestations and Diagnosis

Clinical manifestations of hypertensive encephalopathy are listed in Table 12-6. Severe generalized, sudden headache is a prominent clinical presentation. Neurologic symptoms consisting of confusion, somnolence, and stupor may appear simultaneous with or following the onset of headache. If untreated, progressive worsening of neurological dysfunction occurs, culminating in coma and death. The patient may be quite restless and uncooperative during the initial stages of the syndrome. Other clinical features may include projectile vomiting, visual disturbances ranging from blurring to frank blindness, and transient focal neurologic deficits. Sometimes (especially in children) generalized or focal seizures may be the only clinical presentation.

On physical examination, the blood pressure is invariably elevated (>200/110-120 mm Hg), but there is no certain level of blood pressure above which encephalopathy is likely to develop. The fundi reveal generalized arteriolar spasm with exudates/hemorrhages. Although papilledema is present in most patients with the complication, its absence should not exclude the diagnosis of hypertensive encephalopathy.

When a patient with poorly controlled hypertension presents with severe headache, altered mental status, papilledema, and variable neurologic deficits, the most likely initial diagnosis is hypertensive encephalopathy. A complete but quick evaluation is necessary to rule out other acute neurologic complications of hypertension such as cerebral infarction or hemorrhage and uremic encephalopathy. The only definitive criterion to confirm the diagnosis of hypertensive encephalopathy is the prompt response of the patient's condition to antihypertensive therapy. The syndrome should reverse within a few hours with immediate control of hypertension.

Treatment

The blood pressure should be lowered rapidly to a relatively safe level (over a period of 3-4 hours), but the diastolic blood pressure should probably remain at or slightly above 100 mm Hg to avoid the risk of potential cerebral

---

Table 12-6   Clinical Features of Hypertensive Encephalopathy

• Marked elevation of blood pressure	• Papilledema
• Headache	• Visual complaints
• Nausea, vomiting	• Transient focal neurologic deficits

ischemia. Rapid reduction in the blood pressure produces prompt, dramatic, and significant relief of symptoms of hypertensive encephalopathy. The most important goal of therapy is to prevent permanent neurologic damage. Although potent oral effective agents like minoxidil and nifedipine can control severe hypertension, parenteral drugs such as nitroprusside are preferred in treating hypertensive encephalopathy successfully (16,17). The duration of IV therapy is variable but should be maintained for at least 8-12 hours.

Ischemic Stroke and Intracranial Hemorrhage

Patients with acute stroke and severe hypertension pose a management dilemma. When intracerebral pressure rises as a result of hemorrhage or thrombotic infarction, cerebral blood flow may no longer be under normal autoregulation. Therefore, a reduction in the systemic blood pressure may conceivably compromise the cerebral flow. Conversely, persistence of severe hypertension may resolve spontaneously within 48 hours. There are no definitive data in the literature that provide the practicing physician with a standard approach in managing these patients. At times it is difficult to make a clinical distinction between an ischemic stroke and intracerebral bleed.

With the present state of our knowledge, no firm guidelines can be given about the management of hypertensive crises occurring in patients with cerebrovascular accidents. Based on the pathogenesis of these conditions, especially intracerebral hemorrhage, in the patient with severe hypertension it is advisable to reduce the blood pressure to near-normal levels or to a degree that will not clinically compromise the cerebral function. If there is evidence of progression of the disease or worsening of the neurologic manifestations, then one has to pause and reassess this therapeutic approach. Precautions should be taken to avoid hypotension in these patients, and therefore it is usually advisable not to lower the diastolic blood pressure to less than 100 mm Hg, and to no more than 20% of the baseline blood pressure level.

Acute Aortic Dissection

Clinical Manifestations and Diagnosis

Of the clinical presentations listed in Table 12-7, severe pain is the most important manifestation of acute dissection (18,19). Although it is sometimes confused with pain from other conditions such as acute myocardial infarction, the pain of aortic dissection has certain distinguishing characteristics. For example, the pain of dissection is abrupt in onset and is quite severe right from the onset, whereas patients with acute myocardial infarction rarely report that the pain began abruptly. The pain of myocardial infarction may come and go, whereas aortic dissection pain is constant. It is the quality of pain rather than its precise location that characterizes the patient with acute aortic dissection. Certain descriptions, such as tearing, lacerations,

---

Table 12-7   Clinical Features of Acute Aortic Dissection

- Severe pain in the chest, intrascapular region, neck, midback, sacral area
- Syncope
- Confusional state or headache
- Blindness
- Hemoptysis
- Dyspnea
- Nausea and vomiting
- Melena or hematemesis

---

throbbing, ripping, excruciating, and burning, have been used by patients with acute dissection. Two-dimensional echocardiography, transesophageal echocardiography, computerized tomography angiography and magnetic resonance angiography (MRA) have all been used to diagnose aortic dissection. MRA combined with transesophageal or transthoracic echocardiography yields considerable information; however, MRA is recommended only for patients who are hemodynamically stable and who can be transported to the radiology suite. Digital and/or conventional angiography provides more thorough information concerning the anatomy of dissection and the course taken by the dissection.

Treatment

Once the diagnosis is suspected, immediate medical therapy should be implemented pending the diagnostic tests. Blood pressure should be reduced to near-normal levels with drug(s) that cause the blood pressure to come down smoothly rather than drastically. When instituting medical therapy, one should keep in mind that the force and velocity of ventricular contraction (dp/dt) and the pulsatile flow are important determinants of the shearing force acting on the aortic wall. Attempts should be made to decrease the dp/dt with a suitable drug; whereas drugs that reflex stimulate the heart, such as direct vasodilators, are contraindicated.

Drugs such as trimethaphan, labetalol, and esmolol in combination with sodium nitroprusside have been used in this situation. Trimethaphan, a ganglion-blocking agent, decreases the neural transmission at the myocardial contractility sites and has a negative inotropic effect; therefore, it decreases the pulsative flow and also blunts the sharpness of the pulse wave generated by the heart. Because trimethaphan is not widely available, other therapies should be considered. As already mentioned, other options include labetalol, a combined alpha- and beta-blocking drug, and the ultrashort acting beta-blocker esmolol in combination with sodium nitroprusside.

Acute Left Ventricular Failure

Severe hypertension may precipitate acute left ventricular failure with or without ischemic heart disease; the higher the blood pressure, the harder the left ventricle must work. Decreasing the workload of the failing myocardium can improve the cardiac function. In acute left ventricular failure, myocardial oxygen requirements increase due to increased end-diastolic fiber length and left ventricular volume. This could be particularly undesirable in patients with concomitant coronary artery disease. Prompt reduction of blood pressure with a balanced vasodilating agent such as sodium nitroprusside is indicated. Sodium nitroprusside decreases both pre-load and after-load with restoration of myocardial function and cardiac output. Although the ACE inhibitors, by virtue of their pharmacologic actions, may be useful in this situation, there is paucity of clinical experience concerning the acute therapeutic response in these patients. Diuretics and other standard drugs for acute left ventricular failure should also be used in this setting.

Severe Hypertension Associated with Ischemic Heart Disease

Systemic hypertension increases myocardial oxygen consumption by increasing the left ventricular wall tension. Patients with myocardial infarction and severe hypertension should therefore benefit from blood pressure reduction, but there are no conclusive data to prove that acute treatment is beneficial. Reduction of systemic blood pressure reduces the cardiac work, wall tension, and oxygen demand, and may thus limit myocardial necrosis in the early phase of infarction. With a reduction in the afterload, the hemodynamic status improves significantly in myocardial infarction. Carefully supervised treatment of hypertension in patients with acute myocardial infarction is, therefore, likely to be beneficial.

Pheochromocytoma Hypertensive Crisis

A patient with pheochromocytoma hypertensive crisis may present with striking clinical features. The blood pressure is markedly elevated during the paroxysm and the patient may have profound sweating, marked tachycardia, pallor, numbness, tingling, and coldness of the feet and hands (20). A single attack may last from a few minutes to hours and may occur as often as several times a day to once a month or less.

If pheochromocytoma is suspected, the alpha-androgenic blocking drug, phentolamine, should be given in the dose of 1 to 5 mg intravenously, to be repeated in a few minutes if needed. An alternative to phentolamine would be sodium nitroprusside, but phentolamine is more specific because of its specific mechanism of action. A beta-blocking drug may be useful if the patient has a concomitant cardiac arrhythmia. Administration of beta-blocking agents should always be preceded by either phentolamine or phenoxybenzamine. If this is not done, beta blockade can aggravate the unopposed alpha-mediated peripheral vasoconstriction. Labetalol, a combined alpha- and beta-receptor-blocking drug, has also been advocated for this condition. However, in my experience it is not consistently effective in controlling the clinical manifestations of pheochromocytoma.

Clonidine Withdrawal Syndrome

Abrupt discontinuation of high doses of clonidine may cause a hyperadrenergic state mimicking pheochromocytoma. Clonidine stimulates the alpha-receptors in the brain stem, thus reducing peripheral sympathetic activity. When clonidine is abruptly discontinued (especially high doses) or rapidly tapered, a syndrome has been noted consisting of nausea, palpitation, anxiety, sweating, nervousness, and headache, along with marked elevation of the blood pressure.

Symptoms of clonidine withdrawal can be relieved by reinstitution of clonidine. If there is marked elevation of blood pressure and the patient is experiencing symptoms such as palpitations, chest discomfort, and epigastric discomfort, intravenous administration of phentolamine or labetalol is recommended.

Interaction of Monamine Oxidase Inhibitors and Tyramine

Patients receiving monamine oxidase (MAO) inhibitors are at risk of developing hypertensive crisis if they also take drugs such as ephedrine and amphetamines or consume foods containing large quantities of tyramine. In the presence of an inhibitor of monoamine oxidase, tyramine and indirectly acting sympathetic amines escape oxidative degradation, enter the systemic circulation, and potentiate the actions of catecholamines. Sympathomimetic amines such as those contained in nonprescription cold remedies can also provoke this response. Due to declining use of MAO inhibitors, this reaction is rare.

Cocaine-Induced Hypertensive Crisis

Cocaine use can cause an abrupt, sudden increase in the systemic blood pressure, resulting in a hypertensive emergency. Neurohumoral factors triggered by cocaine likely cause intense vasoconstriction, thus increasing the vascular resistance and the blood pressure level. Sudden rise of blood pressure in a previously normotensive individual may result in a serious cardiovascular complication; the blood pressure should be lowered to safe limits without much delay.

Eclampsia

Eclampsia is a life-threatening cardiovascular complication in a pregnant patient. Although the definitive therapy is delivery of the fetus, the blood pressure should be reduced to prevent neurologic, cardiac, and renal damage. Although other antihypertensive drugs may be effective in reducing the blood pressure, the agent of choice is hydralazine, which has a long record of safety. Methyldopa can also be used in this setting. Animal studies have shown that nitroprusside can cause problems in the fetus; therefore, its use should be reserved for hypertension refractory to hydralazine or methyldopa. The ganglion-blocking drug trimethaphan should be avoided because of the risk of meconium ileus. In pregnancy-induced hypertension, volume depletion may be present and diuretics should be avoided. Intravenous labetalol and hydralazine have been utilized to treat severe hypertension in pregnancy (21). ACE inhibitors and angiotensin-receptor blockers should be avoided due to possible fetal/placental toxicity. Magnesium sulfate is also used as adjunctive therapy to decrease the convulsions.

Prevention

It is very expensive and frustrating to treat complications of severe hypertension, such as stroke, encephalopathy, and aortic dissection. From a pharmacoeconomics point of view, it makes sense to prevent a hypertensive emergency rather than to treat it. Prevention of recurrent hypertensive emergencies is of considerable prognostic significance. Early diagnosis of hypertension and aggressive blood pressure control are critical to prevent hypertensive emergencies.

■   ■   ■

Key Points

- Hypertensive crises are uncommon but should be recognized in order to prevent serious complications.
- Diagnosis of a hypertensive emergency or urgency depends on the clinical evaluation of the patient rather than on a predetermined level of blood pressure.
- Acute rises in blood pressure can cause severe abrupt complications in individuals with even a relatively short duration of hypertension.
- Patients with critical problems related or attributed to hypertension should be hospitalized for appropriate therapy under controlled surveillance and necessary monitoring.
- The choice of oral versus parenteral anti-hypertensive drugs for hypertensive emergencies/urgencies is a matter of clinical judgment based on the patient's cardiac, renal, neurological, and vascular function; the preference for one parenteral drug over another is dictated by the level of target organ damage.
- After the resolution of a hypertensive emergency/urgency, reasons for rapid deterioration in blood pressure control should be evaluated and corrected so a recurrence can be avoided.

■   ■   ■

REFERENCES

1. **Ram CV.** Hypertensive crises. Prim Care. 1983;10:41-61.

2. **Ram CVS.** Diagnosis and management of hypertensive crisis. In: Rippe JM, Irwin RS, Alpert JS, Fink MP, eds. Intensive Care Medicine, 2nd ed. Boston: Little, Brown; 1991:228.

3. **Ram CV.** Management of hypertensive emergencies: changing therapeutic options. Am Heart J. 1991;122:356-63.

4. **Ram CVS.** Hypertensive encephalopathy: recognition and management. Arch Intern Med. 1978;138:1851-3.

5. **Hoshide S, Kario K, Fujikawa H, et al.** Hemodynamic cerebral infarction triggered by excessive blood pressure reduction in hypertensive emergencies. J Am Geriatr Soc. 1998;46:1179-80.

6. **Ram CVS, Boldrick RW, Heller J, et al.** Rapid control of severe hypertension with intravenous infusion of nicardipine: a new therapeutic approach. J Clin Pharmacol. 1989;29:835.

7. **Tumlin JA, Dunbar LM, Oparil S, et al.** Fenoldopam, a dopamine agonist, for hypertensive emergency: a multicenter randomized trial. Fenoldopam Study Group. Acad Emerg Med. 2000;7:653-62.

8. **Oparil S, Aronson S, Deeb GM, et al.** Fenoldopam: a new parenteral antihypertensive: consensus roundtable on the management of perioperative hypertension and hypertensive crises. Am J Hypertens. 1999;12:653-64.

9. **Shi Y, Zalewski A, Bravette B, et al.** Selective dopamine-1 receptor agonist augments regional myocardial blood flow: comparison of fenoldopam and dopamine. Am Heart J. 1992;124:418-23.

10. **Shusterman NH, Elliott WJ, White WB.** Fenoldopam, but not nitroprusside, improves renal function in severely hypertensive patients with impaired renal function. Am Heart J. 1993;95:161-8.

11. **Elliott WJ, Weber RR, Nelson KS, et al.** Renal and hemodynamic effects of intravenous fenoldopam versus nitroprusside in severe hypertension. Circulation. 1990; 81:970-7.

12. **Rubio-Guerra AF, Vargas-Ayala G, Narvaez-Rivera JL, et al.** Comparison between isosorbide dinitrate in aerosol and in tablets for the treatment of hypertensive emergencies. Angiology. 2001;52:131-5.

13. **Ram CVS, Kaplan NM.** Individual titration of didazoxide dosage in the treatment of severe hypertension. Am J Cardiol. 1979;43:627-30.

14. **Bertel O, Conen D, Radu E, et al.** Nifedipine in hypertensive emergencies. Br Med J. 1983;286:19.

15. **Biollaz J, Waeber B, Brunner HR.** Hypertensive crisis treated with orally administered captopril. Eur J Clin Pharmacol. 1983;25:145.

16. **Vidt DG.** Emergency room management of hypertensive urgencies and emergencies. J Clin Hypertens. 2001;3:158-64.

17. **Elliott WJ.** Hypertensive emergencies. Crit Care Clin. 2001;17:435-51.

18. **Garrett BN, Ram CVS.** Acute aortic dissection. Cardiol Clin. 1984;2:227-38.

19. **Ram CVS.** Hypertensive crisis. Cardiol Clin. 1984;2:211-25.

20. **Ram CVS.** Pheochromocytoma. Cardiol Clin. 1988;6:517-35.

21. **Sibai BH.** Treatment of hypertension in pregnant women. N Eng J Med. 1996;335: 257-65.

13

Hypertension in the Elderly

Josh Valtos, MD

Adam Whaley-Connell, DO

Winston Mina, MD

James R. Sowers, MD

Among the geriatric population, typically age 65 and older, hypertension affects more than 60% of the population, requiring global expenditures in the billions of dollars per year (1). Evidence for treating the elderly hypertensive patient has been firmly established. Such treatment reduces overall cardiovascular morbidity and mortality, as demonstrated in multiple trials (2-5). In addition, failure to treat and under-treatment of hypertension increase the risk of coronary artery disease, stroke, dementia, and chronic kidney disease (6,7). The most challenging aspect of treating geriatric hypertension is attaining a significant reduction in systolic blood pressure without adverse effects, which can be disabling, particularly in this population. With the recent release of the JNC-7 guidelines for the treatment of hypertension, much attention has again been directed towards the treatment of the hypertensive elderly patient. As the number of elderly continues to increase, one fact is certain: the number of hypertensive elderly will expand. Numerous studies have demonstrated the enormity of the problem. In particular, the Framingham Heart Study states that the lifetime risk for developing hypertension in a normotensive 55-year-old who lives to age 65 is 90% over the following 20 years (8).

Although the management of hypertension in the elderly can be very complex and requires more frequent monitoring than hypertension in younger patients, multiple studies have demonstrated the benefits of adequately treating elderly hypertensives. Results from the Systolic Hypertension in the Elderly trial (SHEP), the Medical Research Trial (MRC), and the Systolic Hypertension in the Elderly in Europe (Syst-Eur) showed significant reductions in stroke, cardiovascular events, and heart failure (2-4). The MRC trial was a large, randomized, placebo-controlled trial of multiple medications (including amiloride, atenolol, and hydochlorothiazide) in elderly hypertensives. As Table 13-1 demonstrates, the trial clearly established the beneficial effects of treating hypertension in the elderly. In the MRC trial, treating hypertension with either a beta-blocker or a diuretic reduced the rate of stroke by 25% (3). The Swedish Trial in Old Patients with Hypertension trial (STOP) was also a large, randomized trial involving elderly hypertensives, which confirmed the reduction in stroke and cardiovascular disease when treating hypertension in the elderly (5).

In addition, two studies have suggested a reduction in the occurrence of vascular dementia. Although the absolute benefit was small, the Sys-Eur trial showed a 50% reduction in dementia associated with antihypertensive treatment. A recent meta-analysis of studies on elderly hypertensives showed that active treatment reduced total mortality by 13% (95% CI 2-22, $P = 0.02$), cardiovascular mortality by 18%, all cardiovascular complications by 26%, stroke by 30%, and coronary events by 23% (9). Whether treatment focused on diastolic or systolic hypertension, the elderly hypertensive, even older than 80 years, has lower morbidity and mortality with treatment. Table 13-1 summarizes recent trials examining the effects of therapy in the older patient with hypertension.

Pathophysiology of Hypertension in the Elderly

Genetic factors, sedentary lifestyle, obesity, alcohol intake, and dietary salt intake all contribute to the development of hypertension in the elderly, as they do in younger patients. However, there are structural and physiologic changes that occur with aging that explain the high prevalence of hypertension among the elderly.

A predominant factor in the development of hypertension, particularly the traditional concept of isolated systolic hypertension in the elderly, is the gradual stiffening and loss of compliance of the aorta and other large arteries

Table 13-1   Trials Demonstrating the Effects of Hypertension Treatment in the Elderly

Trial (Reference)	N	% Stroke Reduction	% Reduction in Coronary Artery Disease	Congestive Heart Failure	All Cardiovascular Disease
STOP (5)	1627	–47%*	–47%*	–51%	–24%*
SHEP (4)	4736	–33%*	–27%*	–55%*	–32%*
Syst-Eur (2)	4695	–42%*	–26%	–29%	–31%*
MRC (3)	4396	–25%*	–19%	—	–17%*
Syst-China	2394	–38%*	+6%	–58%	–39%

* Represents statistical significance.

(10). This is attributed to the increase in the collagen content and fragmentation of elastin fibers in the large arterial walls, along with deposition of calcium and collagen in the arterial walls (10-12). The decreased compliance results in increased afterload, elevation of systolic blood pressure, and a widened pulse pressure. The elevation of the pulse pressure is due to a pulse wave that is generated by ventricular ejection normally in early diastole, but in the elderly with age associated changes will reach the ascending aorta in late systole. The loss of the pulse wave in early diastole results in a lower diastolic pressure (13), and the resultant widening of the pulse pressure can herald even greater cardiovascular risk.

There is also an increase in peripheral vascular resistance associated with aging. There are many reasons for this. One is atherosclerosis due to the aforementioned collagen deposition and arterial stiffening. Another is the decrease in beta-adrenergic responsiveness of the vascular smooth muscle that comes with aging, causing a decrease in the relaxation of the smooth muscle (10). Coupled with the relatively unchanged alpha-adrenergic responsiveness, this leads to vasoconstriction and increased vascular resistance (16).

Along with the arteriosclerosis that leads to a rising systolic and falling diastolic pressure, there is a progressive dysfunction of the baroreceptor reflexes that is responsible for normal BP changes in posture and activity (17). Not only do barorecepetors play a role in modulating vascular tone, the endothelium also plays an integral role. An intact endothelium produces relaxing factors like nitric oxide (NO) that can affect normal arteriolar tone and blood pressure. The effects of NO are largely unknown on large arteries, but in an animal NO release influenced arterial distensibility (18). With aging, there is damage to the endothelium from atherosclerosis and sheer stress caused by hypertension. The endothelial damage also leads to aggregation of platelets that, in turn, produce the potent vasoconstrictor thromboxane A2. The delicate balance between vasoconstrictors and vasodilators is thus disrupted, with the net result being the predominance of constricting factors. This is another reason why there is an increased prevalence of hypertension in the elderly (16).

Non-Pharmacological Interventions

Lifestyle modifications are an integral part of the treatment of hypertension in the elderly. Both the Joint National Committee and the Society of Geriatric Cardiology recommend lifestyle modification as part of the treatment of hypertension (6,19). Smoking cessation is a mainstay in reducing cardiovascular risk factors associated with hypertension irrespective of age. Elderly smokers with hypertension must be counseled to stop smoking on every visit according to the American College of Physicians. Along with smoking cessation, weight loss and sodium restriction are effective in the treatment of patients with hypertension (20,21).

The Trial of Non-Pharmacological Interventions in the Elderly (TONE) study showed that modest reductions in both dietary sodium and body mass index in the elderly produce significant decreases in systolic blood pressure (20). The trial enrolled 975 persons aged 60 to 80 years with a BP of less than 145/85 and on one medication. The medication was discontinued and the subjects were randomly assigned to one of four treatment arms: sodium restriction, weight reduction, both treatments, or neither. In the end, 44% of the patients in the sodium restriction and weight loss arm managed to avoid hypertension, medication, or cardiovascular events versus 16% of controls. The translation of these results into clinical practice may prove more challenging due to the ability of the researchers to effect and maintain greater behavioral changes than previous studies. The TONE study highlights the effectiveness and feasibility of salt restriction and weight reduction in the treatment of the hypertensive elderly patient.

The Dietary Approaches to Stop Hypertension (DASH) diet also illustrated the effectiveness of dietary interventions as treatment for hypertension (22). Here, 412 patients were randomly assigned to eat a control diet or a DASH diet. The DASH diet emphasizes fruits, vegetables, fish, poultry, grains, nuts, low-fat dairy products, and small portions of red meat, sugar-containing beverages, sweets, and decreased amounts of total and saturated fats and cholesterol. Systolic blood pressure reduction of 8-14 mm Hg was attained by participants utilizing the DASH diet. As a result of these two studies, behavioral and dietary change should be considered an essential therapeutic intervention in the elderly hypertensive patient.

Physical activity has also been advocated as a treatment for high blood pressure. The JNC-7 lists weight reduction to a goal of a normal body mass index (BMI) as a lifestyle modification aimed at managing hypertension (6). BMI is weight in kilograms divided by height in meters squared and stratified into normal (under 25), obese (over 30), and morbidly obese (over 35). Lifestyle modifications may improve antihypertensive drug efficacy, improve cardiovascular morbidity, and in combination may have an additive effect on lowering blood pressure. The main difficulty with increasing physical activity in the elderly hypertensive is adherence to the physician's recommendations. While frustrating, challenging interventions should not be initially dismissed by primary care physicians in favor of pharmacotherapy.

Pharmacotherapy

Medical therapy should be initiated after a fair trial of lifestyle modification has failed to achieve goal blood pressure. Goal BP in the elderly population is defined as less than 140/90 mm Hg or, if diabetes or kidney disease is present, treat to less than 130/80 mm Hg. It is of interest to note that the JNC-7 did not differentiate goal BP based on age. Previously, the JNC-6 had commented on interim goals of systolic BP reduction to less than 160 mm Hg in the elderly population with significant elevated systolic hypertension. This may part from the traditional view of treating isolated systolic hypertension in elderly patients.

Careful consideration of the patient and his or her response to the medication is imperative. Autonomic dysfunction with resultant hypotension affects many elderly, causing postural hypotension, which is a drop in blood pressure. After initiation of pharmacotherapy, frequent visits should ensue until goal blood pressure of less than 140/80 is achieved. In spite of drug therapy, many patients will still have poor control. An epidemiological study in Great Britain by Primatesta et al of elderly adults suggests that more than 67% of older adults should be taking anti-hypertensives, but that only 19% were adequately controlled (140/85 mm Hg) (23). Antihypertensives such as thiazide diuretics, beta-blockers, and ACE inhibitors are considered first-line therapy in the elderly population and will be reviewed as well as other traditional antihypertensives.

Thiazide Diuretics

Many trials have looked at the use of thiazide diuretics as the foundation of antihypertensive therapy. Recently, the Antihypertensive and Lipid-Lowering Treatment to Prevent Heart Attack trial (ALLHAT) looked at ACE or calcium channel blocker versus diuretic to determine the incidence of coronary heart disease in patients with hypertension. The results confirmed that thiazide-like diuretics should be the preferred first agent and at minimum should be included in any multi-drug regimen (24). One major concern of treatment with thiazides is hypokalemia. In the SHEP trial, the benefit of the diuretic group with hypokalemia was lower than the subjects with a potassium greater than 3.5 mg/dL (4). The clinical response should be to provide potassium supplementation or combine thiazides with potassium-sparing diruretics and monitor serum potassium levels. In addition to the antihypertensive benefits of thiazide diuretics, thiazides may also benefit the elderly by reducing the incidence of hip fractures (25).

Beta-Blockers

Beta-blockers have undoubtedly proven their efficacy in elderly patients with a history of coronary artery disease. Even though recent literature has failed to provide convincing evidence that beta-blockers should be a first-line agent in the elderly population, several trials support the benefits of beta-blocker therapy in the elderly, such as the VA Cooperative study group (24,26). The Veterans Affairs Cooperative Study Group on Antihypertensive Agents demonstrated the efficacy of beta-blocker therapy in lowering blood pressure among an older cohort (27). In addition, beta-blockers decrease the risk of stroke and heart failure in hypertensives and reduce subsequent myocardial infarctions in patients with prior coronary events (28,29). The difficulty for many clinicians in adding a beta-blocker to an elderly hypertensive is tolerability.

Most of the adverse effects of beta-blockers in the elderly are a result of their intrinsic activity such as lowering cardiac output and vasodilatation. As a result of the changing pathophysiology of the elderly, beta-blockers should be added at the lowest dose and then gradually titrated to a goal blood pressure the patient tolerates. The starting dose in the elderly is typically about half that used in other hypertensive patients. Because the incidence of renal impairment increases with age, choosing hepatically cleared beta-blockers like metoprolol over renally cleared agents like atenolol is preferred in kidney disease. Additionally, for those elderly hypertensives with concomitant heart failure, cavedilol reduces the risk of death and the risk of hospitalization for cardiovascular cause (30). An important exception to utilizing beta-blockers in a multi-drug anti-hypertensive regimen is the lower response rate of blood pressure control for blacks versus whites (27).

ACE Inhibitors

ACE inhibitors have shown tremendous results, including a reduction in death, for the treatment of hypertension in numerous settings such as myocardial infarction and hospital admission for congestive heart failure (31). Despite favorable data advocating the use of ACE inhibitors, recent data suggests that they are underutilized (32). Although ALLHAT failed to provide sufficient evidence for prescribing ACE inhibitors as a first-line agent, a recent study offered new evidence for elderly hypertensives (24). The Second Australian National Blood Pressure (ANBP2) trial compared cardiovascular outcomes in elderly men who were treated with an ACE inhibitor or a diuretic (33). For men in the ANBP2 trial, using an ACE inhibitor provided superior protection from cardiovascular events and death from all causes.

The differences in the findings between ALLHAT and ANBP2 highlight the difficulties in choosing medication for the elderly hypertensive. When beginning ACE inhibitor therapy, clinicians should start with the lowest dose to avoid side effects. The elderly are particularly sensitive to changes in the renin-angiotensin-aldosterone system, and the risk for first-dose hypotension (or afterload reduction), especially with concomitant diuretic use, is high. Initiation of ACE inhibitor therapy can lead to renal impairment due to decreased perfusion pressure and impaired filtration. Although an initial rise in serum creatinine is expected due to intravacular depletion, one should not observe a greater than 30% rise. Consequently, initially monitoring serum electrolytes is vital for elderly patients on ACE inhibitors.

Angiotensin Receptor Blockers

Although a relatively newer antihypertensive, the angiotensin II receptor blockers (ARBs) have been studied in several large randomized trials and have been well tolerated and effective (34-36). The principle study investigating the effectiveness of ARBs was the Valsartan and Amlodipine for the Treatment of Isolated Systolic Hypertension in the Elderly (Val-Syst) trial. The study was a multicenter, double-blind, parallel-group study. Val-Syst demonstrated that both amlodipine and valsartan effectively lowered systolic blood pressure by 33.4 mm Hg and 33.5 mm Hg, respectively. In addition both medications were efficacious in controlling hypertension in 74.7% of valsartan and 73.0% of amlodipine patients. However, the valsartan group experienced less peripheral edema (26.8% to 4.8%) (36).

Another study, the Losartan Intervention for Endpoint Reduction in Hypertension (LIFE) trial, demonstrated a significant reduction in cardiovascular death and myocardial infarction (37). The primary excretion of ARBs occur through the biliary system, which results in little dosage adjustment for the elderly unless severe hepatic or renal impairment exists. Because the pharmacokinetic properties require little dose adjustment, most ARBs can be prescribed at similar dosages in all age ranges. ARBs block the AT-type 1 receptor and block some of the effects of angiotensin II such as aldosterone release, vascular smooth muscle remodeling, and sodium absorption. As a result, ARBs are often better tolerated than ACE inhibitors, with fewer incidences of cough and first-dose hypotension (38).

Calcium Channel Antagonists

Calcium channel antagonists (CCAs) are also commonly used in the elderly population. As demonstrated in the Syst-Eur trial, long-acting CCAs reduce stroke in the elderly population (39,40). The trial was based on the formulation nitrendipine, but other long-acting agents such as amlodipine, felodipine, or extended-release formulations of nifedipine are available in the United States and are generally recommended. Long-acting agents are used not only for increased compliance but for protection against cardiovascular events such as myocardial infarction, stroke, or sudden death complications that can be associated with shorter-acting agents. In both the International Nifedipine GITS Trial (INSIGHT) and the Nordic Diltiazem trial (NORDIL), the findings supported that CCAs may have more of a preventive effect for stroke versus other cardiovascular outcomes. Both trials compared CCAs against conventional therapy, and there was no difference in outcomes for other major cardiovascular endpoints. CCAs have been used with success in the elderly population (2,41,42). They have also been shown safe and efficacious in patients with advanced CHF in combination with ACE inhibitors, diuretics, and digoxin (Vasodilator-Heart Failure Trial [V-HeFT III]) (43,44). However, care should be given in dosing CCAs because postural hypotension is a potential adverse side effect. Postural hypotension has a higher incidence in the elderly population, so dosing of this particular agent must be titrated; start with the lowest dose and monitor for adverse effects as adjustments are made.

Treatment Approach

With respect to antihypertensive choice, careful consideration must be made to address not only the patient's response to the agent but also the comorbidities of each patient. Initial drug therapy should probably begin with a low dose of thiazide diuretic. If hypokalemia develops, the addition of a potassium-sparing diuretic is reasonable. The majority of patients will fail monotherapy and thereby require the addition of a second agent from a different class such as a beta-blocker, an angiotensin-converting enzyme inhibitor, or an angiotensin receptor blocker. Clinicians should be aware of the adverse effects and additional benefits of antihypertensive medications before determining which agent should be added. A list of comorbid conditions is displayed in Table 13-2, along with specific medications for concomitant treatment of hypertension.

Goal Blood Pressure

According to the recent JNC-7 guidelines, the goal for systolic blood pressure is less than 140/90 mm Hg or less than 130/80 mm Hg for patients with diabetes or chronic kidney disease (6). Although reduction of systolic blood pressure is traditionally the main focus for most clinicians, the JNC made an important distinction by not differentiating goal blood pressure based on age. In the elderly population it is important to recognize the associated mortality associated with reduction of diastolic pressure. Two studies point to the importance of not lowering diastolic pressure too low. The participants in the Rotterdam Study, whose diastolic blood pressure was treated to below 65 mm Hg, had a statistically significant higher risk of stroke (45). Recently, a re-analysis of the data from the SHEP trial demonstrated that even a small reduction in the diastolic blood pressure (5 mm Hg)

Table 13-2   Comorbid Conditions and Specific Medications Recommended for Concomitant Hypertension Treatment

Comorbid Condition	*Drug*
Angina	Beta-blockers
Atrial tachycardia	Beta-blockers
Atrial fibrillation	Diltiazem
Diabetes mellitus	ACE inhibitors
Heart failure	ACE inhibitors, carvedilol
Prostate hypertrophy	Alpha-1 blockers
Renal insufficiency	ACE inhibitors

from antihypertensives caused an increase in the risk of both stroke and cardiovascular events (4,46). It is thus important to note the diastolic pressure upon initiation of therapy and to recognize treatment below 65 mm Hg may represent an increased mortality.

Conclusion

As the population ages, the prevalence of hypertension and its effects will rise. The importance of treating high blood pressure in the elderly cannot be overlooked. Physicians must be cognizant of the major benefits in achieving a lower blood pressure in this group, particularly with the reduction in stroke, heart failure, and overall cardiovascular events. The efforts of physicians can have a large impact on the future financial stability of health care systems by reducing the overall morbidity associated with hypertension in the elderly.

Key Points

- Lifestyle modifications should be part of initial treatment, even in the elderly hypertensive patient.
- Initial pharmacologic therapy of the elderly hypertensive patient should be with a thiazide diuretic, unless a co-existing morbidity favors another antihypertensive class.
- The changing pharmacodynamics of the aging milieu requires initiating medications at a lower dose and titrating upward.
- Multi-drug therapy will likely be necessary and should include a thiazide diuretic; there is no clear choice for a second-line agent for the hypertensive elderly patient but possibilities include beta-blockers and ACE inhibitors.
- Watching the complications of medical therapy such as postural hypotension should be done on every evaluation, and appropriate adjustments should be made.
- Treatment goals should remain the same for the elderly hypertensive as for younger hypertensives; however, diastolic blood pressures should not fall below 65 mm Hg.

REFERENCES

1. **Burt VL, Cutler JA, Higgins M, et al.** Trends in the prevalence, awareness, treatment, and control of hypertension in the adult US population: data from the health examination surveys, 1960 to 1991. Hypertension. 1995;26:60-9.

2. **Staessen JA, Thijs L, Celis H, et al.** Randomised double-blind comparison of placebo and active treatment for older patients with isolated systolic hypertension. The Systolic Hypertension in Europe (Syst-Eur) Trial Investigators. Lancet. 1997; 350:757-64.

3. Medical Research Council trial of treatment of hypertension in older adults: principal results. BMJ. 1992;304:405.

4. Prevention of stroke by antihypertensive drug treatment in older persons with isolated systolic hypertension. Final results of the Systolic Hypertension in the Elderly Program (SHEP). JAMA. 1991;265:3255-64.

5. **Dahlof B, Hansson L, Schersten B, et al.** Morbidity and mortality in the Swedish Trial in Old Patients with Hypertension (STOP-Hypertension). Lancet. 1991;338: 1281-5.

6. **Chobanian AV, Black HR, Cushman WC, et al.** Seventh Report of the Joint National Committee on Prevention, Detection, Evaluation, and Treatment of High Blood Pressure. Hypertension. 2003;42:1206-52.

7. **Prisant LM.** Hypertension in the elderly: can we improve results of therapy? Arch Intern Med, 2000;160:283-9.

8. **Vasan RS, Seshadri S, Larson MG, et al.** Residual lifetime risk for developing hypertension in middle-aged women and men. The Framingham Heart Study. JAMA. 2002;287:1003-10.

9. **Staessen JA, Wang JG, Thijs L, et al.** Risks of untreated and treated isolated systolic hypertension in the elderly: meta-analysis of outcome trials. Lancet. 2000;355: 865-72.

10. **Sowers J.** Hypertension in the elderly. Am J Med. 1987;82:1-8.

11. **Sowers JR.** Effect of advancing age on cardiopulmonary baroreceptor function in hypertensive men. Hypertension. 1987;10:274-9.

12. **Sowers JR.** Norepinephrine and forearm vascular resistance responses to tilt and cold pressor test in essential hypertension: effects of aging. Angiology. 1989; 40:872-9.

13. **Avolio AP, Li WQ, Luo YF, et al.** Effects of aging on arterial distensibility in populations with high and low prevalence of hypertension: comparison between urban and rural communities in China. Circulation. 1985;71:202-10.

14. **Madhavan S, Cohen H, Alderman MH.** Relation of pulse pressure and blood pressure reduction to the incidence of myocardial infarction. Hypertension. 1994;23:395-401.

15. **Benetos A, Rudnichi A, Smulyan H, et al.** Pulse pressure: a predictor of long-term cardiovascular mortality in a French male population. Hypertension. 1997;30: 1410-5.

16. **Hazzard WR.** Principles of Geriatric Medicine and Gerontology, 4th ed. New York: McGraw-Hill Professional; 2003.

17. **Mathias CJ.** Postural hypotension: causes, clinical features, investigation, and management. Ann Rev Med. 1999;50:317-36.

18. **Wilkinson IB, McEniery CM, Webb DJ, et al.** Nitric oxide regulates local arterial distensibility in vivo. Circulation. 2002;105:213-7.

19. **Moser M, Gifford R.** Treatment of High Blood Pressure in the Elderly: A Position Paper from the Society of Geriatric Cardiology. Am J Geriatr Cardiol. 1998;7: 41-42.

20. **Whelton Pk, Appel LJ, et al.** Sodium reduction and weight loss in the treatment of hypertension in older persons: a randomized controlled trial of nonpharmacologic interventions in the elderly (TONE). JAMA. 1998;279:839-46.

21. **Stamler R, Stamler J, Grimm R, et al.** Nutritional therapy for high blood pressure: final report of a 4-year randomized controlled trial. JAMA. 1987;257:1484-91.

22. **Sacks FM, Vollmer WM, Appel LJ, et al.** Effects on blood pressure of reduced dietary sodium and the Dietary Approaches to Stop Hypertension (DASH) diet. New Engl J Med. 2001;344:3-10.

23. **Primatesta P, Poulter NR.** Hypertension management and control among English adults aged 65 years and older in 2000 and 2001. J Hypertens. 2004;6:1093-8.

24. Major outcomes in high-risk hypertensive patients randomized to angiotensin-converting enzyme inhibitor or calcium channel blocker vs diuretic. JAMA. 2002;288: 2981-97.

25. **Schoofs MW, Hofman A, de Laet CE, et al.** Thiazide diuretics and the risk for hip fracture. Ann Intern Med. 2003;139:476-82.

26. **Wink K.** Are beta-blockers efficacious as first-line therapy for hypertension in the elderly? Curr Hypertens Rep. 2003;5:221-4.

27. **Materson BJ, Cushman WC, Massie BM, et al.** Single-drug therapy for hypertension in men: a comparison of six antihypertensive agents with placebo. N Engl J Med. 1993;328:914-21.

28. **Psaty BM, Siscovick DS, Koepsell TD, et al.** Health outcomes associated with antihypertensive therapies used as first-line agents: a systematic review and meta-analysis. JAMA. 1997;277:739-45.

29. **Krumholz HM, Wang Y, Chen J, et al.** National use and effectiveness of beta-blockers for the treatment of elderly patients after acute myocardial infarction. JAMA. 1998;280:623-9. [Erratum in JAMA. 1999;281:37.]

30. **Packer M, Cohn JN, Colucci WS, et al.** The effect of carvedilol on morbidity and mortality in patients with chronic heart failure. N Engl J Med. 1996;334:1349-55.

31. **Flather MD, Kober L, Pfeffer M, et al.** Long-term ACE-inhibitor therapy in patients with heart failure or left-ventricular dysfunction: a systematic overview of data from individual patients. Lancet. 2000;355:1575-81.

32. **Masoudi FA, Wang Y, Havranek EP, et al.** National patterns of use and effectiveness of angiotensin-converting enzyme inhibitors in older patients with heart failure and left ventricular systolic dysfunction. Circulation. 2004;110:724-31.

33. **Wing LM, Ryan P, Beilin LJ, et al.** A comparison of outcomes with angiotensin-converting enzyme inhibitors and diuretics for hypertension in the elderly. N Engl J Med. 2003;348:583-92.

34. **Bulpitt C.** Controlling hypertension in the elderly. QJM. 2000;93:203-5.

35. **Volpe M, Junren Z, Maxwell T, et al.** Comparison of the blood pressure-lowering effects and tolerability of losartan- and amlodipine-based regimens in patients with isolated systolic hypertension. Clin Ther. 2003;25:1469-89.

36. **Malacco E, Vari N, Capuano V, et al.** A randomized, double-blind, active-controlled, parallel-group comparison of valsartan and amlodipine in the treatment of isolated systolic hypertension in elderly patients. The Val-Syst study. Clin Ther. 2003;25:2765-80.

37. **Kjeldsen S, Dahlo FB, Devereux RB, et al.** Lowering of blood pressure and predictors of response in patients with left ventricular hypertrophy. The LIFE study. Am J Hypertens. 2000;13:899-906.

38. **Larochelle P, Flack JM, Marbury TC, et al.** Effects and tolerability of irbesartan versus enalapril in patients with severe hypertension. Am J Cardiol. 1997;80:1613-5.

39. **Pahor M, Corti MC, Foley DJ, et al.** Long-term survival and use of antihypertensive medications in older persons. J Am Geriatr Soc. 1995;43:1191-7.

40. **Psaty BM, Koepsell TD, Siscovick DS, et al.** The risk of myocardial infarction associated with antihypertensive drug therapies. JAMA. 1995;274:620-5.

41. **Hansson L, Lund-Johansen P, Kjeldsen SE, et al.** Randomized trial of effects of calcium antagonists compared with diuretics and beta-blockers on cardiovascular morbidity and mortality in hypertension. The Nordic Diltiazem (NORDIL) study. Lancet. 2000;356:359-65.

42. **Brown MJ, Castaigne A, de Leeuw PW, et al.** Morbidity and mortality in patients randomized to double-blind treatment with a long-acting calcium channel blocker or diuretic in the International Nifedipine GITS study. Intervention as a Goal in Hypertension Treatment (INSIGHT). Lancet. 2000;356:366-72.

43. **Packer M, Ghali JK, Pressler ML, et al.** Effect of amlodipine on morbidity and mortality in severe chronic heart failure. Prospective Randomized Amlodipine Survival Evaluation Study Group. N Engl J Med. 1996;335:1107-14.

44. **Cohn JN, Smith R, Anand I, et al.** Effect of the calcium antagonist felodipine as supplementary vasodilator therapy in patients with chronic heart failure treated with enalapril. V-HeFT III. Vasodilatory-Heart Failure Trial Study Group. Circulation 1997; 96:856-63.

45. **Voko Z, Hofman A, Koudstaal PJ, et al.** J-shaped relation between blood pressure and stroke in treated hypertensives. Hypertension. 1999;34:1181-5.

46. **Somes GW, Shorr RI, Cushman WC, Applegate WB.** The role of diastolic blood pressure when treating isolated systolic hypertension. Arch Intern Med. 1999; 159:2004-9.

14

■   ■   ■

Hypertension in Pregnancy

Maryann N. Mugo, MD

James R. Sowers, MD

ypertension complicates 10% of all pregnancies and is associated with major maternal, fetal, and neonatal morbidity and mortality. Low birth weight in neonates and future hypertension in adult life have all been shown to occur more frequently when abnormal blood pressure persists during pregnancy. Special considerations must be made when caring for pregnant patients with hypertension because prevention of complications is a necessary and achievable goal.

Physiology of Normal Pregnancy

Blood pressure drops normally during the luteal phase of menstruation, and if conception occurs this persists into the early part of pregnancy. The initial change is a decrease in systemic vascular resistance, resulting in peripheral vasodilation and an associated decrease in blood pressure. A compensatory rise in plasma volume occurs progressively throughout pregnancy, with resultant increase in cardiac output (30%-50% up to 16 weeks). The renin-angiotensin-aldosterone system appears to play a role in these changes.

Levels of renin rise throughout normal pregnancy. Several factors contribute to the rise in renin seen in normal pregnancy: estrogen-induced stimulation of renin substrate (angiotensinogen); placental renin synthesis; and compensatory increase due to decreased blood pressure from peripheral vasodilation.

Despite a highly activated renin-angiotensin-aldosterone system (RAAS), normal pregnant patients appear to be naturally resistant to the negative effects of the activated RAAS. Several mechanisms have been postulated to engineer this resistance resulting in protection against the adverse effects of an overactive RAAS. These include downregulation of angiotensin II receptors by the increased levels of angiotensin II; production of prostacyclin and nitric oxide, which antagonizes the effects of angiotensin II; and inherent resistance of the placenta to angiotensin II effects, hence facilitating preferential utero-placental circulation. A disruption of this normal physiology through a number of mechanisms may result in the clinical picture of hypertension in pregnancy. The categories of hypertension in pregnancy are the result of these various etiologies.

Classification of Hypertension in Pregnancy

The classification of hypertension in pregnancy incorporates gestational age, onset of elevated blood pressure, and proteinuria. The clinical relevance of this classification is most apparent in the category with the highest mortality: preeclampsia/eclampsia. This dreaded condition can lead to maternal and fetal mortality if not treated aggressively.

Several classifications of hypertension in pregnancy have been proposed. Both the National High Blood Pressure Working Group on High Blood Pressure in Pregnancy (NHBPEP) and the Seventh Report of the Joint National Committee on Prevention, Detection, Evaluation, and Treatment of High Blood Pressure (JNC-7) have proposed a classification of hypertension in pregnancy (Tables 14-1 and 14-2). The main differences are that in JNC-7 there are five categories as opposed to four in the NHBPEP classification in which "transient hypertension" is categorized as a subcategory of gestational hypertension.

Preeclampsia/Eclampsia

Preeclampsia and eclampsia are part of the same clinical spectrum and are differentiated by the presence of seizures (eclampsia). The pathophysiology of both is identical and may be considered different manifestations or extremes of the same disease. Preeclampsia is a multisystemic syndrome of unknown etiology that presents primarily as hypertension. Other features

Table 14-1   NHBPEP and JNC-7 Categories of Hypertension in Pregnancy

NHBPEP	*JNC-7*
• Chronic hypertension	• Chronic hypertension
• Preeclampsia/eclampsia	• Preeclampsia
• Preeclampsia superimposed on chronic hypertension	• Chronic hypertension with superimposed preeclampsia
• Gestational hypertension	• Gestational hypertension
• N/A	• Transient hypertension

Table 14-2 Description of Hypertension Categories

Chronic hypertension	• BP ≥140 mm Hg systolic or 90 mm Hg diastolic before pregnancy or before 20 weeks gestation • Persists ≥12 weeks postpartum
Preeclampsia	• BP ≥140 mm Hg systolic or 90 mm Hg diastolic with proteinuria (>300 mg/24hr) after 20 weeks gestation • Can progress to eclampsia (seizures) • Specific risk factors (see Table 14-3)
Chronic hypertension with superimposed preeclampsia	• New-onset proteinuria after 20 weeks in a woman with hypertension • Proteinuria and hypertension before 20 weeks gestation • Sudden 2-3-fold increase in proteinuria • Sudden increase in blood pressure • Thrombocytopenia • Elevated AST or ALT
Gestational hypertension	• Hypertension without proteinuria occurring after 20 weeks gestation • Temporary diagnosis (<12 weeks post partum) • May represent preproteinuric phase of preeclampsia or recurrence of chronic hypertension abated in mid-pregnancy • May evolve to preeclampsia • If severe, may result in higher rates of premature delivery and growth retardation than mild preeclampsia
Transient hypertension	• A retrospective diagnosis • BP normal by 12 weeks postpartum • May recur in subsequent pregnancies • Predictive of future primary hypertension

Adapted from JNC-7. AST = aspartate aminotransferase; ALT = alanine aminotransferase.

of this syndrome are diffuse vasospasm, activation of the coagulation system, and dysregulation of hormones involved in the control of blood pressure. Oxidative stress and the inflammatory response may play a key role as well. Table 14-3 lists the risk factors for preeclampsia.

Hemodynamic Changes in Preeclampsia
• ↓ Cardiac output
• ↑ Vascular resistance
• ↓ Circulatory volume
• ↑ Left ventricular mass and end systolic and diastolic volumes
• ↓ Left ventricular ejection fraction
• ↑ Brain and atrial natriuretic peptide
• Renal glomerular dysfunction

Table 14-3   Risk Factors for Preeclampsia

Paternal factors	• Primipaternity • H/o fathering a prior preeclamptic pregnancy • Product of a pregnancy complicated by preeclampsia
Maternal factors	• Primiparity • Teen pregnancy • Young age or older maternal age • History of preeclampsia • Short inter-pregnancy interval • Family history of preeclampsia • Product of a pregnancy complicated by preeclampsia • Oocyte donation
Underlying/chronic disorders	• Chronic HTN • Renal disease • Insulin resistance • Low maternal body weight • Factor V Leiden; protein S deficiency • Antiphospholipid antibodies • Hyperhomocysteinemia
Environmental factors	• Stress, work, and emotional strain • Inadequate diet • Smoking
Pregnancy related factors	• Multiple pregnancy • Urinary tract infection • Congenital anomalies (structural) • Hydrops fetalis • Hydatidiform mole • Chromosomal abnormalities

Adapted from Dekker G, Sibai B. Primary, secondary, and tertiary prevention of pre-eclampsia. Lancet. 2001;357:209-15; with permission.

What we see clinically in preeclampsia are the late manifestations of a cascade of events. The initial triggering factor remains to be elucidated, but it seems to be of placental origin. Proposed mechanisms include genetic disorders such as thrombophilic tendencies and immunological mechanisms.

Clinical Manifestations of Preeclampsia/Eclampsia
- Epigastric and right upper quadrant pain
- Headaches, seizures, and visual disturbances
- BP at or greater than 160 mm Hg; systolic at or greater than 110 mm Hg diastolic
- Cardiac decompensation
- Retinal hemorrhages
- Intrauterine growth retardation

- Oliguria
- Proteinuria greater than 3 g/24 hr (associated with increased serum albumin levels)
- Increased serum creatinine greater than 2 mg/dL
- Platelet count less than 100,000/mm³ with or without micro-angiopathic hemolytic anemia.

Clinical Approach to Hypertension in Pregnancy

The management of hypertension in pregnancy begins with pre-pregnancy assessment of blood pressure status, evaluation for secondary causes, and delineation of any end organ damage. If already hypertensive and blood pressure management is considered, treatment should be initiated with medications known to be safe during pregnancy (Table 14-4). The approach to treatment also depends on initial presentation. If the patient presents with chronic hypertension, for instance, the approach will be different from that of preeclampsia/eclampsia.

Measurement of Blood Pressure

The International Society for the Study of Hypertension in Pregnancy (ISSHP) has provided the following guidelines for blood pressure measurement in its ISSHP Statement:

- The pregnant woman should be seated with feet supported for 2-3 minutes.
- An appropriately sized cuff should be used.
- Systolic and diastolic blood pressure should be recorded with the diastolic read as the Korotkoff 5 (disappearance), and Korotkoff 4 (muffling) only utilized when a phase 5 is absent.
- Bilateral blood pressure should be checked at first visit, and if any significant difference is detected, the right arm should be used thereafter. Significant differences require referral to an expert.

Table 14-4   Preferred Drugs for Chronic Hypertension in Pregnancy

Drug	Safety	Dose
Methyldopa	Long-term studies and use show safety and efficacy	250-500 mg daily in 2 doses
Labetalol	Safe; reduced side effects (compared with beta-blockers)	200-1200 mg in 2-4 doses daily
Beta-blockers	Generally safe but may cause intrauterine growth retardation	Depends on agent

Measurement of Proteinuria

The ISSHP Statement has also provided guidelines for proteinuria measurement:

- Urinalysis (dipstick) should be a guide for further testing because it has a high rate of false positives and false negatives. On dipstick, 1+ (30 mg/dL) is often but not always associated with 300 mg/day or higher proteinuria.
- Abnormal proteinuria is most likely when measured in a timed collection over 24 hours; greater than 300 mg/day is abnormal for pregnancy.
- Spot urine protein/creatinine ratio 30 mg protein/mmol or higher creatinine is an alternative that is superior to qualitative analysis (dipstick) and equivalent to 24-hr urine collection.

Treatment of Hypertension in Pregnancy

Chronic Hypertension

The approach to treatment is based on maternal and fetal risk outcome potential. Lifestyle modification within safe limits (avoid excessive weight loss and exercise) is the first choice. Salt restriction to 2-4 g/24hr may be incorporated, although no data exists on the benefits of this. Choice of antihypertensive medication is based primarily on safety. Lower blood pressure results in fewer infants who are small for gestational age. If severe chronic hypertension is not treated in the first trimester, fetal losses as high as 50% will occur primarily due to superimposed preeclampsia. Pregnant hypertensive patients should be strongly advised against smoking and drinking.

Limited data exist on the use of calcium channel blockers and clonidine. Diuretics may be used if the other preferred drugs cannot be used. Angiotensin-converting enzyme (ACE) inhibitors and angiotensin receptor blockers (ARBs) are contraindicated in pregnancy due to their risk of maternal uterine ischemia and fetal renal dysgenesis.

Preeclampsia and Eclampsia

Treatment of preeclampsia may be pharmacological or non-pharmacological. The pharmacological treatment is shown in Table 14-5.

Sodium nitroprusside may be used only if the other medications fail. The dose is 0.25 μg/kg/min to a maximum of 5 μg/kg/min. Fetal cyanide poisoning may occur if used for more than 4 hours, and especially in the third trimester of pregnancy.

Magnesium sulphate is used primarily for treatment of seizures. It may be synergistic with calcium channel blockers in causing hypotension, so caution should be used if these two medications are used concurrently.

Table 14-5   Pharmacological Treatment of Preeclampsia

Medication	Dose/Route	Onset of Action	Adverse Effects	Comments
Hydralazine (first-line)	5 mg IV bolus then every 20-30 minutes to a maximum of 25 mg; repeat in several hours	IV 10 min IM 10-30 min	Headaches, flushing, tachycardia, arrhythmias, nausea, vomiting	Drug of choice
Labetalol (second-line; may also be first-line)	20 mg IV bolus, then 40 mg in 10 minutes; 80 mg every 10 minutes for two additional doses to a maximum of 220 mg or IV drip of 1-2 mg/min until desired effect, then reduce to 0.5 mg/min	5-10 min	Flushing, nausea, vomiting, tingling of scalp	Drug of choice
Nifedipine (controversial)	5-10 mg PO; repeat in 30 min as necessary to max 30 mg	10-15 min		When used with MgSO$_4$, may cause hypotension

Non-Pharmacological Treatment

Delivery of the fetus is the definitive therapy for preeclampsia. Immediately after emergency delivery, the risk of seizures, abruptio placentae, thrombocytopenia, cerebral hemorrhage, and multi-organ failure decreases dramatically. Consideration of fetal maturity may delay delivery but only in selected cases. Delivery may also be delayed until blood pressure is reasonably controlled and fluid and electrolytes have been stabilized in certain cases. If seizure occurs, immediate delivery of fetus by cesarean section is indicated.

Postpartum Care

If a patient has chronic hypertension, medication postpartum should be continued as needed. All anti-hypertensive medications considered safe in pregnancy may enter breast milk; however, these are in very low concentrations. The American Academy of Pediatrics considers beta-blockers and calcium channel blockers compatible with breastfeeding. Labetalol and propranolol have the least concentration in breast milk. Nifedipine and verapamil may be alternatives if beta-blockers are contraindicated. Diuretics may reduce milk volume and also suppress lactation, so they should be avoided. ACE inhibitors and ARBs are contraindicated during lactation. Counseling should be given to women who were hypertensive during pregnancy regarding the possibility of long-term cardiovascular risks. If their hypertension was transient, the risk for hypertension in future pregnancies should be addressed.

In patients with preeclampsia, post-delivery monitoring is paramount. Medications should be adjusted as the blood pressure improves. Peripartum cardiomyopathy may complicate normal pregnancy or pregnancy complicated by hypertension. Fulminant nephrosclerosis occurring postpartum has been described, which is characterized by oliguric renal failure and severe hypertension.

■ ■ ■

Key Points

- Hypertension in pregnancy causes maternal and fetal morbidity and mortality.
- When identifying hypertension in pregnancy, gestational age, onset of hypertension, and proteinuria are determining factors. Other factors such as secondary hypertension and end-organ damage are considerations.
- Preeclampsia/eclampsia is responsible for most of the mortality associated with hypertension in pregnancy; identification is imperative for emergency therapy.
- Lifestyle changes such as salt restriction, low-impact exercise, and smoking and alcohol cessation are integral components of care.
- Labetalol and methyldopa are the safest antihypertensive medications that can be used in pregnancy; ACE inhibitors and ARBs are contraindicated in pregnancy.
- Post-partum care includes adjustment of safe blood pressure medications to meet blood pressure goals and discussion of potential risk of future cardiovascular complications.

■ ■ ■

REFERENCES

1. The Seventh Report of the Joint National Committee on the Prevention, Detection, Evaluation, and Treatment of High Blood Pressure. NHLBI; NIH. August 2004.
2. National High Blood Pressure Education Program Working Group Report on High Blood Pressure in Pregnancy. NHLBI; NIH. July 2000.

3. **Kaplan NM, Lieberman E, Neal W.** Hypertension with pregnancy and the pill. In: Kaplan's Clinical Hypertension, 8th ed. Philadelphia: Lippincott Williams Wilkins; 2004.

4. The Classification and Diagnosis of the Hypertensive Disorders of Pregnancy: Statement from the International Society for the Study of Hypertension in Pregnancy. Hypertens Pregnancy. 2001;20:ix-xiv.

5. **Saudan PJ, Brown MA, Farrell T, Shaw L.** Improved methods of assessing proteinuria in hypertensive pregnancy. Br J Obstet Gynaecol. 1997;104:1159-64.

6. **Beardmore KS, Morris JM, Gallery EDM.** Excretion of antihypertensive medication into human breast milk: a systematic review. Hypertens Pregnancy. 2002;21: 85-95.

Index